"Dame Cicely Saunders, nurse, physician and founder of the modern hospice movement once said, 'You matter because you are you, and you matter to the end of your life. We will do all we can not only to help you die peacefully, but also to live until you die.' In *Counselling and Psychotherapy with Older People in Care*, Felicity Chapman puts life into these words. Her 'out of the box' approach to psychotherapeutic work with older adults is a refreshing and much-needed text which infuses a strong interest in the lived narrative. This area of health care has not received the attention, nor the research, that it deserves. Felicity's contribution redresses this oversight and offers a rich, practice-informed account. It provides strength to the delivery of evidence-based practice for this cohort while calling for a more nuanced approach that is not diagnostic or disorder focused. Readers are led on a journey of belief that older people in care still have much to teach and share and deserve to be provided with opportunities to work through a variety of psychological issues. This book provides clinicians with a manual filled with real-life accounts that are honest and heart-warming. It is to be commended to anyone who cares about the wellbeing of older adults."

– Julianne Whyte, OAM, CEO and Founder of the Amaranth Foundation

"In *Counselling and Psychotherapy with Older People in Care*, Felicity Chapman sets out to excite and equip psychotherapists across disciplines to create spaces of hope and re-invigoration for ageing populations in care. Her book is a must-read guide! By sharing stories of her psychotherapeutic work with seniors such as Harold, we are invited into the complexities and challenges of the work as well as being introduced to evidence-based practice and practice-based evidence. The detailed account of relevant psychological approaches offers a breadth of perspective. The illuminating personal stories of the elderly and the meticulous unpacking of work within residential care systems are written with rigor, elegance and humor and make for compelling reading."

– Shona Russell, mental health social worker and
Co-Director of Narrative Practices Adelaide

of related interest

Positive Psychology Approaches to Dementia
Edited by Chris Clarke and Emma Wolverson
Foreword by Christine Bryden
ISBN 978 1 84905 610 6
eISBN 978 1 78450 077 1

Developing Excellent Care for People Living
with Dementia in Care Homes
Caroline Baker
ISBN 978 1 84905 467 6
eISBN 978 1 78450 053 5

Person-Centred Counselling for People with Dementia
Making Sense of Self
Danuta Lipinska
ISBN 978 1 84310 978 5
eISBN 978 1 84642 892 0

Anti-discriminatory Practice in Mental Health Care for Older People
Edited by Pauline Lane and Rachel Tribe
ISBN 978 1 84905 561 1
eISBN 978 0 85700 947 0

Person-Centred Dementia Care, Second Edition
Making Services Better with the VIPS Framework
Dawn Brooker and Isabelle Latham
ISBN 978 1 84905 666 3
eISBN 978 1 78450 170 9

COUNSELLING
— AND —
PSYCHOTHERAPY
— WITH —
OLDER PEOPLE
— IN CARE —

A Support Guide

Felicity Chapman

Jessica Kingsley *Publishers*
London and Philadelphia

The list on page 56 is from SEVEN STRATEGIES FOR POSITIVE AGING by Robert D. Hill. Copyright © 2008 by Robert D. Hill. Used by permission of W. W. Norton & Company, Inc.

First published in 2018
by Jessica Kingsley Publishers
73 Collier Street
London N1 9BE, UK
and
400 Market Street, Suite 400
Philadelphia, PA 19106, USA

www.jkp.com

Library of Congress Cataloging in Publication Data
Names: Chapman, Felicity, author.
Title: Counselling and psychotherapy with older people in care : a support guide / Felicity Chapman.
Description: Philadelphia : Jessica Kingsley Publishers, [2018] | Includes bibliographical references.
Identifiers: LCCN 2017032047 (print) | LCCN 2017044179 (ebook) | ISBN 9781784507510 (ebook) | ISBN 9781785923968 (alk. paper)
Subjects: LCSH: Older people--Care. | Older people--Counseling of. | Psychotherapy for older people.
Classification: LCC HV1451 (ebook) | LCC HV1451 .C624 2018 (print) | DDC 362.6/6--dc23
LC record available at https://lccn.loc.gov/2017032047

British Library Cataloguing in Publication Data
A CIP catalogue record for this book is available from the British Library

ISBN 978 1 78592 396 8
eISBN 978 1 78450 751 0

Printed and bound in Great Britain

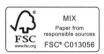

for Marjorie

Contents

APPENDICES

Acknowledgements

To my husband Peter Chapman for keeping the cogs of our "home machine" well-oiled when I was lost in "book land" and for being supportive in many other ways.

To our two boys Ethan and Tyler for living with the third child – my writing. (And maybe you are right. Perhaps I really am a master gamer in disguise with those screens!)

To friends Mark O'Donoghue, Tina Stothard, Pooja Sawrikar, Sigrid Heuer, Pouya Baniasadi and Kathy Drillis for encouraging my writing endeavours and a big thank you to Anne-marie Taplin for her sharp editorial eye.

To former colleague Bronwen Paine who was my original "partner in crime" – fellow explorer and practitioner in psychotherapeutic work with older adults in care. And to all past and present team members who have worked with me in aged care across organizations.

To Dr Greg Smith and Dr Jaklin Eliott from the Graduate Program in Counselling and Psychotherapy at the University of Adelaide. If it weren't for the opportunity to present the inaugural lecture on Counselling Seniors in 2015 – which allowed me to arrange my thoughts – then none of this may have eventuated. So inspired was I by aged care being included as something of value that the initial draft of this book was written in a month after sharing with students! And to the students of this lecture who, over the years, have nourished me with their insight and interest.

To those who gave feedback on earlier drafts: Dr Greg Smith, Dr Nicol Moulding and Janine Barelds – psychotherapists I admire greatly – and to my father Jeff Hudson and step-mother Jan for their encouragement.

To Professor Nancy Pachana of the school of psychology at the University of Queensland and coordinator of the Ageing Mind

Initiative for her enthusiastic support and unwavering passion for promoting the psychological and emotional wellbeing of older adults. Also for agreeing to review this book in its entirety and offering her expertise to refine it.

To Julianne Whyte OAM, PhD candidate, mental health social worker and CEO of Amaranth Foundation for also reviewing this book in its entirety and giving me invaluable feedback and support.

To all specialist reviewers for how generous they were with their time and whose thoughtful responses I appreciated immensely. I felt humbled and excited to be "standing on the shoulders of giants". Listed from A to Z by first name:

- Ms Andrea Gregory, psychologist (clinical) and clinical lead at Northern Health Network: on palliative work, Cognitive Behavioural Therapy and pain management.

- Dr Cate Howell CSM, OAM, general practitioner, psychotherapist, lecturer and director of Dr Cate Howell & Colleagues: on grief, Cognitive Behavioural Therapy and Interpersonal Therapy.

- Dr Elizabeth McHugh, clinical geropsychologist at CHE Senior Psychological Services: on the whole of Chapter 6.

- Dr Emma Hanieh, clinical psychologist, director of The Adelaide ACT Centre, senior lecturer University of Adelaide: on Acceptance and Commitment Therapy.

- Ms Krystie Edwards, mental health social worker and certified sensorimotor psychotherapist at the Adelaide Trauma Centre: on trauma management.

- Ms Shona Russell, mental health social worker, teacher, family therapist and co-director at Narrative Practices Adelaide: on Narrative Therapy.

To my peer supervision group: Helen Fincher, Janine Barelds, Lynn Lobo and Vanessa Hounslow who quietly go about transforming the lives of their clients. They also energize me with their belief that therapeutic encounters cannot live by technique alone, that when we connect with our whole being, the world can be a better place.

To the Adelaide Primary Health Network and the Northern Health Network, thank you for valuing the psychological and emotional health of seniors by continuing to offer the Residential Wellbeing programme.

To Jessica Kingsley Publishers for picking this project up and being so helpful during the journey to publication.

Last, but by no means least, to all older people in care whom I have had the privilege to consult and learn from over the years.

Preface

Have you ever felt the relief of knowing that your world was somehow all right again? A flood of appreciation for the good things in life after feeling long dragged down by a sickness or hardship? And even if your external circumstances were not looking up, this relief was about knowing that you were not alone? A spiritual awakening perhaps, a friend to be with, a good deed shown, a change of heart? This realization bringing a new perspective? You could now do this thing called life: face the challenge and reap the reward?

Did everything around you appear just that little bit more shiny? Did your warm glow on the inside sometimes burst into a smile? And if you were not always interested in sporting a toothy white grin, or even had a sense of euphoria, do you remember feeling something very different inside? No longer distress and despair, but peace and hope? Life could now go on?

This transformation is what I often see in my work as a psychotherapist with older adults. It might be as big as a radical improvement in mood, or as small as a subtle change in their look as you witness someone feeling noticed and heard, seemingly for the first time. Sometimes these transformations are reflected in quantifiable outcomes. At other times they are fleeting glimpses of relief not easily captured, not easily turned into a statistical picture. Whether these transformations are measurable or not – what matters to me is that these "conversations with purpose" have been meaningful for that person – offered healing no matter how small. Their wife still may have died, they may no longer be able to walk, or their stroke may have rendered their once able body into a group of uncooperative parts, but they are standing taller (even for a moment) on the inside. "Thank you," they might murmur with quiet appreciation, "I don't think anyone has ever listened to me like that before." Or, "It means the world to me," if they have just been asked what it means to talk in this way.

One client, in particular, embodied for me this transformation. Her name was Mary, and she was 91 when I first entered her room. She had a major fall just days after moving into a new residential facility. It was the worst one she had ever had. It had damaged her body but, worse, it had sent her confidence spiralling. So scared was she now of falling again, or dissolving in panic in front of others, that she had cocooned herself in her room where fear and self-recrimination began to feast on her mind in silence.

"I've always been so positive!" she implored to me that first day, her face contorted with embarrassment and despair. She listened patiently, but eyed me suspiciously, when I told her about staff feeling concerned and how our programme could help. It was clear that she knew little about counselling, but enough to see it as a threat. As Mary sat stiff and sore on her floral chair, with her hallmark colour of purple dancing all around the room, I could see that she was in a dilemma. Would she feel more like a failure being involved in this counselling thing – likely to just highlight her weaknesses – or more alienated than ever before from an identity of positivity if she tried battling on all by herself? Would she mind giving it a go, I asked. "I don't know," she said. Reluctantly, she agreed but much later confessed, "I really wasn't sure about this at first."

Yes, I could see that, the fear. It was the same look I see in countless others of her vintage. They have survived the Depression and World War II (for goodness sake), surely they can get through this? "I'll be all right," they will say with a tear in their eye. "When times are tough, the tough get going!" they joke, and you know your presence and offer of help smells to them like defeat. And when you use the words "counselling" and "wellbeing", they look at you like a budgie has just done its business on your head. "What's the point of talking?" You can hear them think, "I just need to grit my teeth and bear it like I have done with everything else. Young ones these days..."

You see, rarely would a person in their eighties or nineties be familiar with the concept of counselling or psychotherapy, much less value it, and even more unlikely: *ask* for it. Think about it, they were in their thirties and forties already when Aaron T. Beck developed Cognitive Therapy. Cognitive Behavioural Therapy was not even a term that had been coined! And now, they might know of Freud, but anything related to *that* sort of help is synonymous with being one of *them*. "I'm not crazy!" they will assert. And they are right.

So, there Mary was, struggling with a wish to be as polite as she could but also aiming to protect any semblance of self-respect that she had left. By session three, as rapport developed and she got a taste for feeling heard, we started to speak about depression and what she had noticed. Her score on the Geriatric Depression Scale (GDS) was 20 out of 30 indicating the presence of debilitating symptoms. This knowledge, much as it resonated with her, also seemed to encourage a fresh wave of hopelessness – about herself and the counselling process. "But what else can you expect at my age?" she asked. "Depression is not a normal part of ageing," I countered. "What about we just put our toe in the water for a few more sessions and see after that? But, of course, you can say you don't want to continue at any time," I responded, trying to balance hope with her right to decline.

She continued, and was adamant not to take any anti-depressants. In the coming months, little by little, she began to explore more deeply her concerns and was one of the most open seniors I have met in how she embraced an exploration of various modalities. She investigated her thought, feeling and behaviour cycles, practised mindfulness and self-compassion, learnt how to get space from unhelpful thoughts, identified her strengths, shared her story, re-positioned herself against the problem, and partook in experiments where she compared predictions with actual experience. I suspect that she was a natural born scientist as she appeared to relish such exploration, but desire to succeed was as much of a blessing as it was a curse. As much as it motivated her to persevere, it also "beat her up" – something that we often needed to address.

As with any sustainable growth, it was two-steps-forward-and-one-step-back. But at session number 19 we reviewed her progress. The results shocked her (and me). Despite having had another fall, not taking the anti-depressants recommended to her by her doctor and experiencing some intervening family challenges, her post score for the GDS was an astonishing *2* out of 30. And, at our final session – the twentieth one – she summarized her experience of a year in therapy by writing, "An amazing journey from a deep hole of despair and hopelessness, not wanting to live, to a life well worth living with bonuses. [I now] have more confidence and self-worth."

But, when I left to say goodbye, what struck me – more than her GDS score or feedback – was her smile. Her face looked alive, her eyes twinkled in the dimly lit room, and her body (better, but not fully recovered) rested comfortably in her chair. I knew then that her sunset years were now a whole lot better.

Mary was unique. She was as sharp as a tack, could speak easily, could hear and communicate well, could see, write and was highly motivated. While this combination is rare, it is the experience of therapy for those who, like Mary, are in their eighties and nineties that colour the pages of this book. But it is not just their experience that I would like to share with you. I would also like to share with you how the process of providing psychotherapy has taught me more about what it means to be relevant and respectful with this group. It has challenged me to consider the wider context, and helped me develop a practice that is deeply satisfying.

People's sunset years may not always be filled with laughter, but they can be a place where peace and happiness reside. Working as a psychotherapist with older adults may not always be easy, but it can be a place of rich reward. And though ageism still wafts through our community like an unpleasant odour, building senior-friendly frameworks across care systems is critical for the promotion of positive ageing. How these things might be possible is the subject of this book.

INTRODUCTION

Ever since working as a care attendant in my early twenties at an aged care facility, the concept of exploring lives rich with experience has appealed to me. After a shift I wondered about the iceberg of a life I had attended to that day. What parts of themselves did they still relate to as a much younger version stared back in a wedding photo on their wall? Who were they before they forgot their name or could no longer get out of bed? Who were they even now as death waited for them at the door?

But there was no time for these investigations in the course of a busy shift. It was all bodies, dressing and routine. And god forbid if your resident was late for lunch – the kitchen staff would put *you* out on the menu! It is ironic that the very desire that had me leaving aged care – to study counselling instead of feeling straitjacketed by the machine of physical care – is the same one now that has me listening to a resident in their room.

Back then, in 1991 in Australia, the idea of counselling seniors had not even occurred to me. While the Council on the Ageing had been established for three decades and, in the United States, clinical geropsychology had been a field of practice for almost 20 years,[1] psychotherapy for seniors was not a subject covered in either my counselling diploma or Lifeline training. At least my social work degree recognized our ageing population but no job opportunities were available that married counselling with ageing and end of life issues.

So it was with a full-circle sweep that, decades later, I found myself in a mental health unit with a new programme aimed at improving the emotional and psychological functioning of older people in care who were mostly over 80. There were few, if any, guidelines. There was no session limit, vague eligibility criteria and no need for a mental health care plan from a doctor. My colleague and I were wide eyed and neither of us had training in geropsychology theory or practice. But, between us, we had decades of counselling experience and I was strongly influenced by Narrative Therapy. We then set about having faith in the process of being client centred and consulting the real experts – the older adults themselves.

Looking back I treasure this time of exploration and learning. More than ever before it taught me to train my attention on the person in front of me and, while many times I felt uncertain, overwhelmed or frustrated, I kept coming back to one thing: my interest in their story. While I was not familiar with geropsychology or gerontological theory at the time, I consider this original consultation process more valuable than any learning I have done since from "the giants" in this field. Why? Because it caused me to think "outside the box" and not approach work with this population in a way that is often synonymous with mainstream psychology or the medical model.

Counselling and Psychotherapy with Older People in Care is an appreciation of all that the field of geropsychology has to offer but it is also a gentle challenge. Through a practice-informed perspective I invite you to look beyond the frame of medicine or science – beyond mainstream psychology – and consider a philosophy and practice that is at times in contrast to traditional approaches. This slightly alternative approach is a fusion of my practice knowledge, my interest in Narrative Therapy philosophy and "third wave" psychological practices, as well as more traditional evidence-based practices. Perhaps this whirlpool of ideologies could be seen as embracing the art and science of psychotherapeutic practice with older adults? It is where "Rogerian psychotherapy" meets "the medical model", where the qualitative and the quantitative both share centre stage and where best practice is both "evidence-based practice" and a reflection of "practice-based evidence".

Most of us are familiar with the term "evidence-based practice" but Professor Anne Swisher (2010) explains how "practice-based evidence" is gaining traction in the medical community. She suggests that too much emphasis is given to cause and effect models of enquiry and says:

> to quote Albert Einstein, surely one of the greatest scientific minds in history: *"Not everything that can be counted counts and not everything that counts can be counted."* In the concept of Practice-Based Evidence, the real, messy, complicated world is not controlled. Instead, real world

practice is documented and measured, just as it occurs, "warts" and all. It is the process of measurement and tracking that matters, not controlling how practice is delivered. (Swisher 2010, p.4)

Therefore, in terms of psychotherapy with older adults, I believe that both best practice models should be entertained: evidence-based practice and practice-based evidence. While this book does not share research using the practice-based evidence model, it is still interested in sharing an orientation that favours "practice wisdom". Valuing this orientation also opens the space to be informed by disciplines other than clinical psychology. To date, the definition of best practice is strongly related to psychological research which uses an evidence-based practice model in how it rates an intervention or approach. As a mental health social worker and sessional lecturer for those studying a graduate counselling and psychotherapy university course it excites me to imagine how other disciplines might join the discourse on best practice for clinical work in the aged care sector through practice-based evidence research models or practice wisdom.

Counselling and Psychotherapy with Older People in Care aims to be clinically relevant while still offering an alternative approach. It aims to be inclusive by appreciating skill sets and orientations that sit both within and outside the discipline of clinical psychology and mental health social work. This book is also interested in sharing with you the voices that told me what mattered – the product of my consultation with clients over the years. The product of seeking to understand how seniors would like to be defined and engaged with. These pages yield within them a desire to share and add to the current knowledge base, to inspire and challenge, to educate and sustain an interest across disciplines about what it means to work therapeutically with a thought-provoking and diverse group of people – seniors.

But who is a senior? It is difficult to pin down an exact age definition as it depends on whether a country is developed or not and, if it is, what the pension eligibility is for that country. In Australia, where I am from, the age pension requires people to be 65 and over so I will use this as my definition of "older adult". Of course, whether someone *feels* old is an entirely different matter. This is more related to individual and social perceptions of ageing – and the comfort level our society has with the concept of being old – which is discussed later in this book.

So we have arrived at a yard stick to determine who is an older adult but, as with young people, there are important categories to define each sub-group. Consider the difference between a just retired 65-year-old to a long retired 90-year-old. One might be ready to travel the world and the other might be content with a cup of tea and a chat. To be in step with modern gerontology I will associate the "young-old" with people aged between 65 and 74 years of age, the "old-old" with those between 75 and 84 years of age, and the "oldest old" with those 85 and over (Pachana 2016, p.16). In relation to the "oldest old" I have a term of my own: "advanced senior". I believe that it has an air of reverence to it, like acknowledging seniority in the workplace. For the purposes of this book I will refer to all of the above as either "senior" or "older adult". Aside from simplicity, this is also because whenever I have asked my clients how they would like to be described – "the elderly", "the aged", "older adults" or "seniors" – they have always chosen the last two.

When it comes to trying to define "old age" beyond the amount of years one has lived, there are many variables to consider. Where children grow according to a fairly uniform set of developmental increments, the same cannot be said for the experience of old age. While, according to Erik Erikson's Stages of Psychosocial Development theory, someone in the maturity stage (65+) may well be reflecting on and questioning their life, individual experience of the ageing process can vary enormously. Have you seen the movie *Still Alice*? I thought it was a very touching account of how Alzheimer's disease can affect the young – in this instance a woman who had just turned 50. At the other end of the spectrum, a person may be a centenarian but still have their health (and sense of adventure) as the book *The Hundred-Year-Old Man Who Climbed Out of the Window and Disappeared* (Jonasson 2015) delightfully portrays.

The many variations on the experience of "ageing" are exactly why gerontologists distinguish between four distinct categories of the ageing process. The categories are: *chronological age*, how many years you have lived; *biological age*, the state of your physical and neurological health; *psychological age*, how you interpret your world and any changes to cognition, personality and ability to adapt; and *social age*, the changing nature of the roles you adopt in intimate and broader social contexts (Hooyman and Kiyak 2011). While some of these categories might overlap or affect each other, the fact is that you can have "young-old" people in more limiting circumstances than the "oldest old" and vice versa.

The perfect storm

Now that we know who we are talking about when we use the word "senior" we can turn our attention to what is happening in the lives of these older adults. As I write this section I have to admit to you – it is a little overwhelming. Why? Because the issues *are* overwhelming. Not only is there a high incidence of distress amongst our senior population, and the numbers of them grow by the day, but there are not enough psychotherapists coming forward to meet this need and not enough training or support for these practitioners. And that is just the tip of the iceberg! It is a perfect storm. But I hope that by the end of this book you can see what elements are needed to create more calm conditions, how you can play your part in this change, how you might feel more supported, and why you might become totally addicted to working with this wonderful group of people. As Steve Jobs once said: "the only way to do great work is to love what you do" (in Chowdhry 2013).

Incidence of distress

Between 2008 and 2012 the Australian Institute of Health and Welfare conducted a study to look into the incidence of depression in residential care facilities. It was, and still is, the largest analysis of its kind in that country. What it discovered was breathtaking:

> More than half (52%) of all permanent aged care residents at 30 June 2012 had symptoms of depression, as did 45% of people admitted for the first time to residential aged care between 2008 and 2012. These are likely to be underestimates... (Commonwealth of Australia 2013, p.24)

Researchers of this study relied on an automatic intake process for all new residents – the Aged Care Funding Instrument. This instrument is needed to rate the level of individual need and decides how much the facility should be paid by the government for that person's care. It includes a mood assessment called the Cornell Scale for Depression

(CSD) which is viewed as a reliable screening tool to identify depressive symptoms in people with cognitive impairment and/or for seniors.

The report, entitled *Depression in Residential Aged Care 2008–2012*, applauded the ability of mandatory residential intake processes to identify the presence of depressive symptoms and suggested that being able to use this process to intentionally measure mood might lead to more effective management of psychological health. But the peppy undertones of hope in how this process could alert doctors to the potential need for a medication increase seemed at odds with what was blaring loudly in my ears: a large proportion of seniors are experiencing symptoms of depression and there was no discussion about how psychotherapy might be used to address this need.

Results from this study rang true for me though. I thought of the many times I have watched as depression wafted around the face of an older client. Both in aged care facilities and in the community, I remembered how soul destroying experiences of sorrow, dysphoria and chronic grief can be: a World War II veteran deeply ashamed of himself, a great-grandmother staring despondently out the window, a woman who used to love adorning her hair with a brightly coloured clip no longer wanting to groom herself or even get out of bed.

Yes, depression is real amongst seniors and can be so subtle that it is easily undetected. The older adult, their family and the professionals who care for them are more likely to address issues of physical concern – a gammy leg, an infection, eye problems – or practical matters like personal care assistance at home or food quality in a facility. The Australian Psychological Society (APS) also points to the problem of depression being underreported in our senior population. For the current cohort of older adults, who appear uncomfortable seeking help about issues related to the psychological, the APS suggests that they "may be more likely to describe their experiences in physical rather than emotional terms" (APS 2000, p.18). This position paper goes on to identify the following as major mental health problems experienced by older people:

dementia, anxiety disorders (e.g., generalised anxiety disorder, panic attacks, post-traumatic stress disorder, and agoraphobia), mood or affective disorders (e.g., major depression and bipolar disorder), and substance use disorders (abuse of alcohol or prescription drugs such as minor tranquillisers (benzodiazepines)). Psychotic illnesses such as schizophrenia, delusional disorders, and paranoia are less common.

Other mental health problems that may affect older adults include adjustment and sleep disorders. (APS 2000, p.18)

The results of both the Depression in Residential Aged Care report and the APS position paper are both disturbing and illuminating as they point to a great need in the psychological health of older adults. However, if the incidence of major mental problems is of concern – and even then likely to be underreported – then the grumblings of general distress or dysphoria are in greater proportion and all the more overlooked. My observation is that experiencing change on a grand scale, living with persistent pain, experiencing loss and grief, and losing independence and control contribute to broader unmet need. Indications of this might not register on any clinical measurement but if you ask, "Have you not felt yourself lately?" or "A lot of people who go through similar changes as much as that can feel a bit overwhelmed, worried or flat. I was wondering, is this the case for you?" then you might be given access to a world where life as they knew it has vanished into thin air. Silent distress – fear, frustration, sadness, shock, shame – are large rocks that they keep stumbling over.

Our ageing population

It is no secret that we have an ageing population. In the United States one in five will be 65 or older by 2030, by which time the population of those in this age group would have nearly doubled since 2000 (Transgenerational Design Matters 2017). The population of those 65 or older in England and Wales increased by almost one million from 2001 to 2011 (Office for National Statistics 2013, p.2) and there are strong concerns that health and care systems are not ready for this rising tide (Age UK 2017). Over in Australia, the number of 85-year-olds will increase from 0.4 million in 2010 to 1.8 million by 2050 (Commonwealth of Australia 2011a, p.xxvi). The United Nations reports that:

The increasing proportions of aged persons have been accompanied, in most populations, by steady declines in the proportion of young persons... In the more developed regions, the proportion of older persons already exceeds that of children; by 2050 it will be double. (United Nations 2002, p.15)

It is not a skateboarding teenager that you will need to look out for while taking a stroll outside but a lycra-clad grey bike enthusiast or a speeding mobility scooter!

Everyone appears to be either scrambling to make a dollar – appealing to the "grey" market – or save a dollar – protecting against gloomy economic forecasts. Interests and policies may differ depending on which part of the globe you live on or which side of the political fence you sit. But if you are living in a developed country, no matter what your geographical location or personal view, the fact is that our population is ageing.

In short, the logic appears to go – if it is a problem now then it is only likely to become a bigger one in years to come; better to try and tame the beast now before it grows in strength. Have you noticed, as you drive around your neighbourhood, an increase in retirement villages being built? Have you heard the pleas in the media to address "the aged care crisis"? Implicit in all these efforts are concerns about our ageing population. It is like a dust storm that our society is bracing itself for. Whether we realize it consciously, or have it float around in our unconscious, the issue of our expanding cohort of seniors seems to be the salt with which everything else is flavoured. You hear about a campaign to raise awareness about elder abuse. "Yep," you think, "because if we don't address that now, it will only get worse." You read up about developments in end of life planning – advanced care directives – and the whisper around your ears is "…because the more seniors we have, the more this will become an issue". It is like "our ageing population" is at the end of every sentence when we think about issues related to older adults, the economy or end of life care.

But just as we seem to be facing this reality, there are also signs of an intriguing desire to avoid it. We want to talk about feeling young, not growing old. "Fight the signs of ageing!" advertising slogans suggest; and we do. Is it that interest in anything "old" is the antithesis of our Western culture? In Chapter 8 we will consider this broader social context of ageing but, for now, it is enough to be aware that responding to an ageing population might illuminate a deep and diverse set of values about ageing. These values seep into everything, and the field of psychotherapy is no exception. It can affect how interested practitioners are in working with older adults, how much governments are willing to spend on creating job opportunities in this area, and the extent to which specialist training courses are available.

As in many things, it is hard to tell which comes first – the chicken or the egg. But whatever the complex set of reasons, one thing is clear: supply is not meeting demand.

Shortage of worker interest and expertise

In 2008 Nancy Pachana, then Associate Professor of Clinical Psychology at the University of Queensland, described the number of Australian psychologists who work in long-term care facilities as "bleak"(Pachana 2008, p.8). Five years on and she was concerned that a vast majority of psychologists in Australia are still not heeding the call to work in facility settings, and that this workforce crisis is evident in other countries around the world (Pachana 2013).

In an *In-Psych* article about training for work in aged care, the authors challenged, "How many psychologists that you know have provided a professional service in an aged care facility this year? How many people do you know with grandparents, parents, or other relatives living in a nursing home? Our crystal ball," they wryly pointed out, "predicts that for the great majority of readers, the answer to the second question is a notably larger number than the response to the first one, to which the answer is likely to be zero" (Helmes, Bird and Fleming 2008, p.12).

Their question sounds like the beginning of a joke, "How many psychologists does it take to change a light bulb in an aged care facility? None. There won't be any. Go find a nurse." But it is no joke. The lack of psychologists, psychotherapists and social workers in long-term care settings is a problem, especially given what we know about the incidence of distress. The above article goes on to suggest, "There are many reasons few psychologists provide services in residential care. One of the main reasons, however, is that few psychologists have the interest, skills, or the applied experience to assist individuals…" (Koder and Helmes 2006, in Helmes *et al.* 2008, p.2). The authors then urge for a stronger ageing component in traditional postgraduate clinical training along with more supervised clinical placements. They conclude that, "It is clear that demand far exceeds current supply and that experienced supervision for work in aged care facilities needs expansion" (p.2).

I would say a resounding, "Hear, hear!" and believe that psychotherapists from a range of backgrounds should heed the call into work with seniors: mental health social workers, nurses, occupational therapists and accredited counsellors. Just as in psychology, numbers in other professions are low. For example, only 0.6 per cent of mental health social workers have indicated aged care as their primary field of practice (Australian Association of Social Workers, personal communication, 2016)[2].

I also agree that more training opportunities are needed, especially in Australia. There are postgraduate and certificate courses (centre based or online) available specific to psychological intervention with seniors. However, as alluded to earlier, such options are mostly defined by philosophies linked to mainstream psychology. As an example of a move toward more choice of industry training, in 2015 I was delighted to deliver an inaugural lecture on counselling seniors in a postgraduate psychotherapy programme through the University of Adelaide. This inclusion was as much of a celebration as it was a sad reminder of just how slow our learning institutions are in prioritizing aspects related to ageing.

Given the already high incidence of distress, the ageing population and the possibility that Baby Boomers will be more receptive to counselling (demand it even)[3] than older generations, it makes sense to expand this specialist field as wide as possible. But surely in doing so we need to also expand the terminology to include a range of professionals who have chosen to specialize with seniors? In the United States if you are not a geropsychologist you could complete postgraduate training and become a "geriatric counsellor" – a rather unfortunate title in my opinion. We use the term "psychotherapist" to include a range of disciplines and training levels – so why not design a term that denotes this specialist area but is also inclusive? What about *gerontological psychotherapist*? As a mental health social worker who specializes in gerontological work, that is what I now call myself.

As suggested above, interest and expertise in psychological work with older adults in is a water hole that still looks rather dry in some parts of the world. There are precious droplets of hope forming though. You are one of those – you would not be reading these lines if you did not have some interest in this work. And, as the following suggests, you are not alone. Momentum is gradually building and it is my hope that this book adds to a collective experience of moving forward. Instead of a dry dust storm, I hope we soon have many "ponds" in the sector filled to overflowing.

Same ripple, different ponds

We, as a global society, are recognizing how important it is to value and care for older adults. This is evidenced by the International Day of Older Persons, established by the United Nations in 1990, and the International Association of Gerontology and Geriatrics, founded in 1950. We have the *Journal of Gerontology: Psychological Sciences* which is distributed worldwide and psychotherapy with older adults has been a research topic for around eight decades (Knight 2004).

In Australia it is heartening to know of a range of materials that address the psychological and emotional wellbeing of older adults. The work of beyondblue – Australia's leading online resource for depression and anxiety – is one example. Their 2009 campaign Over Bl**dy Eighty! collated stories from the over-80 group on how they led physically and mentally healthy lives; the handbook *What Works to Promote Emotional Wellbeing in Older People* (Wells *et al.* 2014) was designed to support aged care staff; and their factsheets or booklets on "Older People and Depression" or "Dementia and Depression" are important resources for older adults, their families and related carers or professionals.

There are also best practice resources such as the *Guidelines for a Palliative Approach for Aged Care in the Community Setting* (Commonwealth of Australia 2011b) and key position papers have drawn attention to the twin issues of mental health and older adults. First, the Australian Psychological Society published *Psychology and Ageing* (APS 2000) and then the Australian Association of Social Workers released a paper four years later entitled *Improving Service Responses for Older People with a Mental Health Condition* (AASW 2014). All these resources, as well as the establishment of the Psychology and Ageing Interest Group in 2001, are indicators of a growing interest in supporting the health needs of older adults.

For best practice guidelines in psychotherapeutic work with seniors the ripple extends across the developed world. There are guidelines for Australian practitioners (Pachana, Helmes and Koder 2006) but these draw heavily on what is perhaps seen as the "global gold standard" which are those formulated for psychologists in the United States (American Psychological Association 2014, 2017). Here, there are 21 guidelines which the following lists in relation to each heading:

1. "Psychologists are encouraged to work with older adults within their scope of competence."

2. "Psychologists are encouraged to recognize how their attitudes and beliefs about aging and about older individuals may be relevant to their assessment and treatment of older adults, and to seek consultation or further education about these issues when indicated."

3. "Psychologists strive to gain knowledge about theory and research in aging."

4. "Psychologists strive to be aware of the social/psychological dynamics of the aging process."

5. "Psychologists strive to understand diversity in the aging process, particularly how sociocultural factors such as gender, race, ethnicity, socioeconomic status, sexual orientation, disability status, and urban/rural residence may influence the experience and expression of health and of psychological problems in later life."

6. "Psychologists strive to be familiar with current information about biological and health-related aspects of aging."

7. "Psychologists strive to be familiar with current knowledge about cognitive changes in older adults."

8. "Psychologists strive to understand the functional capacity of older adults in the social and physical environment."

9. "Psychologists strive to be knowledgeable about psychopathology within the aging population and cognizant of the prevalence and nature of that psychopathology when providing services to older adults."

10. "Psychologists strive to be familiar with the theory, research, and practice of various methods of assessment with older adults, and knowledgeable of assessment instruments that are culturally and psychometrically suitable for use with them."

11. "Psychologists strive to develop skill in accommodating older adults' specific characteristics and the assessment contexts."

12. "Psychologists strive to develop skill at conducting and interpreting cognitive and functional ability evaluations."

13. "Psychologists strive to be familiar with the theory, research, and practice of various methods of intervention with older adults, particularly with current research evidence about their efficacy with this age group."

14. "Psychologists strive to be familiar with and develop skill in applying culturally sensitive, specific psychotherapeutic interventions and environmental modifications with older adults and their families, including adapting interventions for use with this age group."

15. "Psychologists strive to understand and address issues pertaining to the provision of services in the specific settings in which older adults are typically located or encountered."

16. "Psychologists strive to recognize and address issues related to the provision of prevention and health promotion services with older adults."

17. "Psychologists strive to understand issues pertaining to the provision of consultation services in assisting older adults."

18. "In working with older adults, psychologists are encouraged to understand the importance of interfacing with other disciplines, and to make referrals to other disciplines and/or to work with them in collaborative teams and across a range of sites, as appropriate."

19. "Psychologists strive to understand the special ethical and/or legal issues entailed in providing services to older adults."

20. "Psychologists strive to be knowledgeable about public policy and state and federal laws and regulations related to the provision of and reimbursement for psychological services to older adults and the business of practice."

21. "Psychologists are encouraged to increase their knowledge, understanding, and skills with respect to working with older adults through training, supervision, consultation, and continuing education."

When Medicare lifted its restrictions in the States in 1990 it meant that older adults could finally be reimbursed for accessing psychological services and the mental health industry for older adults began to flourish. For example, CHE Behavioral Health Services, which provides psychological and psychiatric support to residents in long-term care settings, started as a small family-owned business in 1995 and has now grown to an enterprise servicing over 700 facilities and related settings nationwide (CHE Behavioral Health Services 2017).

Between reimbursements from the government and insurance companies, the provision of psychology services in the States is attractive to both facilities and residents with neither having to pay out of pocket expenses in most instances. And with regulations requiring facilities to provide alternatives to the use of psychotropic medications and restraint, interest in psychological services is now greater than ever. The Netherlands also has a well-developed system of care for older adults by making available "nursing home psychologists" (Pachana 2008). Other countries are not quite as supportive of ensuring that residents have access to specialist mental health services though. For example, at the time of writing, Australia still excludes residents of facilities from accessing Medicare-funded treatment by accredited psychologists and mental health social workers through its Better Access to Mental Health Care programme, but pressure to reform this legislation is mounting (Council on the Ageing 2017).

Many "ponds" around the world are emerging with an interest to provide counselling and psychotherapy to older adults. Some are fuller than others. But, even where legislation is restrictive, there is acknowledgement that our ageing population – whether in the community or in care – need subsidized or free access to mental health services so their psychological and emotional wellbeing can be maximized.

This book aims to add to the widening ripple that is psychotherapy with older adults. While there are a growing number of practitioners speaking about their work with seniors[4] I believe that there is room for more. The greater the number of voices, the more likely it is that enthusiasm for this area will grow. And the more diversity of voices – extending beyond the discipline of clinical geropsychology – the greater potential there is to attract a variety of skills and expertise that can only add a richness to service delivery.

If you have an interest in psychotherapeutic work with seniors then this book is the guide to cheer you on – to give you a practice-informed perspective on common issues and support in overcoming challenges. It is a compliment to the academically rich and medical model-focused material available. This information is important – by all means be familiar with it – but if it has your eyes feeling a little heavy then I hope this book injects you with a fresh surge of motivation and confidence. Motivation and confidence that the aged care sector so desperately needs.

A special breed of senior

Harold lies in the darkened room with curtains drawn. It is 1:30 in the afternoon and his lunch tray seems to almost sigh at the untouched food. His words are soft and not many. He listens, looking down, as you speak about concerned staff referring him to a counselling programme – you are here to see if he is interested. "I'm fine," he says, in a rare attempt to meet your eye, and it is clear to you that he is not. He is 88 years old and five months ago his right leg had to be amputated due to complications with diabetes. Immediately after, he was transferred to an aged care facility an hour's drive from his wife Elizabeth, two years his senior, who could no longer care for him at home. A month after that he was transferred to this facility; his wife can now more easily visit him. But, he tells you, he does not know why she bothers. "There's no point," he says, and you wonder if he is also referring to being alive.

Your time allocation is running out; you need to decide what to do next. You suspect depressive symptoms, critical even, but other than suggesting to staff a review of medication you are not sure if Harold would engage in therapy – even admit that there is a problem. Can you help him? Should you even try? He hasn't said "no" to you but it is possible that at any moment a wall of refusal might squash any hope of helping him further. What is your duty of care: to respect the signs of disinterest and leave or continue to engage?

But would he even let you assess him? How can you provide psychotherapy to someone who is giving all the messages to be left alone?

To many, this scenario might sound like the idiom you-can-lead-a-horse-to-water-but-you-cannot-make-him-drink. But has the horse been successfully led to the water hole yet? Has Harold enough information and experiential understanding to make an informed decision about whether counselling might benefit him or not? He is already on the maximum dose for an anti-depressant – would psychotherapy even be advisable?

At what point might you decide that he really is not interested? In what instances would continuing to engage be imposing and disrespectful and when could withdrawing be a grave case of lost opportunity based on either rigid therapeutic protocols or therapist anxiety? How would you arrive at client goals if he has not come to you with a problem? Quite the contrary – he is suggesting to you that he is fine. How could intervention navigate his other co-morbidities of diminished sight, minimal hand dexterity, emerging short-term memory loss, along with other cognitive presentations such as difficulty with concentration? Of this last point, you wonder if this difficulty has more to do with natural ageing and fatigue (perhaps remedied by an earlier time slot), with depression, pain or neurological decline. Perhaps a combination of all four?

Yes, people over 85 in a long-term care context are a special breed of older adult. It is true, we must avoid stereotyping the advanced senior and reject negative assumptions about age. There are many advanced seniors who live healthy and happy lives despite the losses that can present themselves as chronological age moves on. Some may be living in the same family home as they have done for decades, others may have moved into an independent living retirement village, others may be in and out of hospital and still others may have needed to enter a long-term care option.

As is the case in the wider community, psychological support is not needed by everyone. But that does not mean that we should avoid campaigns to encourage good mental health like ones instigated by the Mental Health Foundation, Mental Health America or SANE Australia. If encouraging help-seeking behaviour and having sufficient resources to respond skilfully to mental health issues in the wider community is important, then it is all the more important for our ageing population. The current cohort of advanced seniors, especially, have been acknowledged as particularly stoic and not likely to consult a mental health professional (APS 2000). Their unique disposition is the subject of Chapter 2 where sociological research will shed light on the challenges of psychotherapeutic engagement.

However, if skill and sensitivity are required to engage effectively with the current cohort of advanced seniors, then this is even more the case for those who reside in long-term care facilities. First, they virtually never self-refer. Even advanced seniors in the community who present themselves to therapy, largely due to the insistence of others, can have a sense of self-directed interest in improving their wellbeing. And most would have had to agree in some fashion to having a referral processed if therapy is to be subsidized.

It is commendable indeed that government-run psychotherapy programmes for seniors in care exist, as they do in Australia, and have a wide funnel of intake. However, this means that initial contact can look much like an involuntary (or at least uninitiated) scenario common to how children or young adults might enter therapy. And as I have mentioned earlier, despite a growing availability of specialist resources for psychotherapy with seniors, interest and expertise is minimal. This is no truer than in relation to work with advanced seniors. Case scenarios about working effectively with the oldest old are hard to come by.

If therapists can engage effectively with advanced seniors in long-term care – a special breed of senior – then they are also likely to do so for those who are more voluntary or ones who are younger and may be more receptive to therapy. Knight (2004, p.254) even goes so far as to say that psychotherapy for seniors in long-term care should be considered, "a *sub*speciality within clinical geropsychology" (emphasis mine). Now, you might not want to narrow your expertise to this extent, but this statement does underscore just how unique psychotherapy is in the context of an aged care facility.

I believe that if you can develop understanding and confidence in the facility setting, then you have already climbed Mount Everest! Other adventures are not likely to seem as challenging. However, the focus here will not be to the exclusion of other contexts. Other cohort-specific challenges will be considered along the way, and you will also have the opportunity to reflect on what is relevant to you in the "personal reflection" at the end of each chapter. Placing a spotlight on advanced seniors in long-term care facilities is not designed to limit your skill base but broaden it. It also pays homage to a population of adults who confess to me that they feel cut off from society, ignored; "thrown away" is how one lady put it to me just yesterday. But before we investigate this context further, first, a disclaimer.

A disclaimer

In presenting to you a practice-based resource on engaging older people in psychotherapy I would like to emphasize that the contents of this book are my considered opinion born more of experience than training. Certainly, I am trained and accredited in the field of mental health but I do not possess any qualifications that relate to geropsychology. What you have in these pages are my reflections, which have not been subjected to the rigours of research that hold within them a burning desire for worker integrity.

Some of these reflections resonate with or extend what others in the field of geropsychology are saying; other reflections are alternative opinions. My opinion is only one voice. What is more important to me is that many voices in this field emerge. Your experience and voice is one of those. Whether you agree or disagree with what I present, for me, that is irrelevant. What I hope, more than anything, is that as you read my considered opinions you will be taken further in your own journey of thought and practice with seniors.

Finally, I would like to note that my experience sits within a context of short- to medium-term intervention – through either a salaried position or private work – within the Australian health care system and in relation to the nuances of Australian culture. In both instances my role has been to support those who are able to show some sort of progression in a psychotherapeutic context. In my country, we have specialized services for those whose care needs are more psychiatric in nature or more related to neurological impairment such as in the case of Alzheimer's. Both the Older Persons Mental Health Service and the Dementia Behaviour Management and Advisory Service are, respectively, available nationally and are a key resource to address distress that is not likely to ease without non-medical intervention, ongoing support or environmental changes within the facility.

Unlike a geropsychologist I am not required to be conversant with a range of medical terminology, pathology or design interventions for staff to assist in behaviour management. But as a psychotherapist interested in working with older adults, I see it as my duty to have an adequate knowledge base of assessment tools normed for this population, common co-morbidities and effective response strategies. Some of this knowledge has been gained through research, some through "on the job" learning and some through the learnings of life. While I understand the importance of knowing my professional limitations, as a familiar face in a facility I am often the first person with whom senior staff discuss experiences of resident distress. Sometimes I refer, and other times my recommendations alone appear to resolve the issue. The advice in this book is based on my experience with older adults, family and facility staff and is of a general nature. It should not replace individual consultation with a supervisor or mental health professional for a specific issue.

PART 1

THE CONTEXT

CHAPTER 1

RESIDENTIAL LIVING

Have you ever stepped inside a long-term care facility? What sights, sounds and smells come to mind? They are places that many try to avoid. "He doesn't much like coming here," a resident might say of her son. Why? "Because he hates the whole lot. I have to say, I can understand what he means," she says with a rueful look.

Love them or hate them, they are places where many live. They are often a bustle of unceasing activity, a maze of corridors and pin codes. Some rooms can have hold-your-breath aromas that change your mind about lunch. "Help! Please help!" a resident may call out as you pass, and others stare blankly at the television. There is death, there is life. Some staff truly care, some not so much. Each facility has its own culture and way, which can often change depending on who is sitting at the helm. But no matter what colourful mix of the pleasant, unpleasant or neutral, working in them and with them is what psychotherapy for residents of long-term care is all about.

Building trust with staff

If you are a counsellor or psychotherapist for older people in care then you need to work very hard at building knowledge and faith in your service. Why? Because these relationships are central to your referral base. Facility staff are intricately connected to the resident and also their trust in you can significantly affect how supportive they will be of your recommendations. You need to be able to "sell" the benefits of psychological care as just as an important part of wellbeing as physical care. Perhaps more than for any other population, physical and mental health are two sides of the same coin. But care staff are often not aware of how challenging behaviours and psychological distress are so inextricably linked. Staff training is outside the scope of this book but I have developed resources which I have used one on one and in group settings to educate facility staff and increase their skill in managing resident distress. It can take effort and time to get the message across – with high turnover in staff a little hurdle to jump – but building yourself as a trusted resource for staff formally and informally can be well worth it in my experience. This is especially true if you need to take a firm stand on an issue, which is what the next section explores.

Who is your client?

Services that are limited to individualized models of care, such as through a mental health care plan which is the main mode of accessing subsidized psychological support in Australia, make it all the more challenging to effectively address distress when it bleeds into a wider system such as the family. I fondly remember my days as the social worker/counsellor for the Multiple Sclerosis Society because of the freedom I had in taking a multi-systemic approach to emotional and psychological health. It did not matter if I was conducting individual, couple, family, group therapy or running carer retreats – the focus was exploring the impact and facilitating healing *for all*.

The question "who is your client" can relate to a number of dimensions: the guidelines of the programme or the organization you are working in, who is paying for the service, issue complexity, or personal and professional ethics. Sometimes others (staff, doctor, family) are more distressed than the senior, sometimes concerns are symptomatic of deeper issues (conflicting agendas, grief, family tension), and sometimes the "problem" may be more to do with staff wanting compliance than anything else.

None of this probably surprises you. If you have been a psychotherapist for any length of time (or even just have a few years under your belt) you will know with certainty that human relationships are fascinating if not a little infuriating at times. So many different agendas, communication styles, personalities, histories, health needs, resources and challenges. It really is a wonder that we mostly get along! But, of course, like a courtroom judge, the therapist is exposed to times when things are not going so well. If life is normally a knotty tangle of relationship need, then why should old age be any different? Long-term care facilities are like shrink-wrapped country towns where relationship dynamics are intensified – for better or worse – and there is also the delicate issue of dependency.

Taking a holistic approach to "who is your client" affords you a clearer picture of every terrain, every referral. If it is within your role then spend time with stressed staff exploring options, role model and teach reflective listening skills, have couple or family sessions with the resident (with their consent), offer individual appointments to a distressed wife or son. But keep at the focus – the centre of all you do – the rights and wellbeing of the senior. For, ultimately, they are your client. The following scenario and set of response options sheds light on how multi-faceted questions around "who is your client" can be.

Mrs Grout was referred to you because staff were becoming exhausted with her complaints and demands. Family were also feeling exasperated and stressed by her pleas to return home.

1. *Staff and family are the client.* Mrs Grout is not at all bothered by *her* behaviour. She considers it completely justified. Everyone else is the problem in her opinion. You discover from family that she has always been a glass-half-empty sort of person. Why should now be any different? You support staff and family dealing with a person who does not appear interested in changing but you do not continue with therapy for the resident on the grounds that it would be a violation of client consent: she does not want to see you.

2. *Everyone is the client.* You learn from Mrs Grout that she is done with being nice. She was in a domestic violent marriage for decades and now, at the ripe old age of 90 and with nothing to lose, wants to be free to optimize her wellbeing. You counsel her on how she might go about this without sabotaging her ultimate desire and you counsel others on how they might create boundaries to protect staff and not compromise equity for other residents.

3. *The senior is the client.* After empathizing with Mrs Grout you suspect that there are deeper issues behind her behaviour. She is grieving: for the loss of independence, choice, control, her changed body and life. Getting to

the heart of the matter and informing staff of her dilemma (only with her permission) she learns to heal and be more considerate while staff learn to be more understanding.

4. *Everyone is the client.* You learn from family and staff that Mrs Grout's personality has changed in the year she has been at the facility. You observe her memory, logic and lucidity to be "patchy" – sometimes it appears normal and others times it does not. You also observe that she appears to have no insight into the impact of her actions on others. You suspect that she has an unusual dementia presentation that, if diagnosed accurately, could help staff and family develop different expectations and responses (Mrs Grout is not being mean and neither are others if they do not react each time to her calls – Mrs Grout is not able to keep score). You recommend a psycho-geriatrician assessment.

Perhaps an even more contentious issue is proceeding with psychotherapy if others appear more distressed than the senior. Seniors – especially ones in facilities – can be very vulnerable. Maybe they appear interested in therapy because they are scared of what might happen if they do not participate? Maybe conducting therapy is colluding with notions that the senior is the problem when, really, it is more systemic than that. Knight (2004) presents a poignant example of how staff became annoyed because depressed residents were now cured and becoming too assertive! Could the psychotherapist fix this "problem" please?

Long-term care facilities are like any other organization; they want life to run smoothly. Compliance and efficiency can be agendas that are at odds with a genuine interest in wellbeing for the senior: one that promotes individuality and independence. I am afraid that there are no easy answers to this, but being aware of this minefield is critical if you are to try and navigate through it. Later, we will consider the question of "whose problem is it" in more detail as it relates to determining suitability for therapy. Next, we will continue exploring the need to work as effectively as possible within the constraints of facility living.

Negotiating the space

This section is divided into two parts: negotiating the organizational-political space, and negotiating the literal physical space.

The organizational-political space

As alluded to earlier, long-term care facilities each have their own culture and way of operating. What to do when this is at odds with your understanding of wellbeing, or even if it violates a code of conduct or is an instance of abuse?

As you round the corner to see your next client, Mr Childs, you hear the cooing voice of a carer attending to him. You tap on the slightly open door to let them know of your presence. "Won't be long!" Cherie the carer calls chirpily, and you take your place in the hall while she busies herself with the task of helping Mr Childs back from toileting. Mr Childs had a stroke two years ago, making his speech slurred and one half of his body droopy. Patiently, you have listened to him for the last three sessions and have learnt of his career in architecture, love of fine wine and admired his clever wit. He has been struggling with depression but making some advances. Your attention tunes back to the noises inside Mr Child's room – "There's a boy!" you hear Cherie declare. "Don't want the waterworks to get out of control now, do we?!" she adds, evidently helping him clean up his face. She exits with a bright smile and says loudly to you, "He's a bit teary today, love. Might need an extra box of tissues!" She laughs, and walks off down the corridor.

I happen to not think of seniors as "boys" or "girls". They are adults. And I appreciate it when issues of emotional sensitivity are treated, well, sensitively. But if I addressed every act that I believed transgressed my view on dignity, not only would I have no energy left to work with clients but I would have got a large number of staff off-side along the way. Sometimes, as they say about life, "you have to choose your battles".

While not every less-than-ideal encounter can or should be taken up with management, there are matters that are more of a priority. This is no more the case than with allegations of abuse or suspected abuse because, as the slogan goes, "there is no excuse for elder abuse".[5] There is no clear-cut way through this territory; it is largely up to the discretion of the individual. In Australia, for example, there are no mandatory reporting laws requiring people to report suspected elder abuse, unless they are facility staff. Even in the facility context, however, the mandatory requirements do not cover any or all instances of elder abuse. Staff are only required to report allegations in relation to "...unlawful sexual contact or unreasonable use of force... [but] for other incidents of alleged abuse [at the hands of staff or others]... the law assumes adults can make their own decisions, about whether or not to do anything about the abuse that they experience" (Aged Rights Advocacy Service 2017). For psychotherapists working with older adults either in the community or in care, the role is to offer confidentiality, information about their rights, freedom of choice and support to take the steps that they wish – if they wish to.

The complexities around if, when and how to respond to allegations of abuse are numerous. For example, many older adults often don't want to "bite the hand that feeds them", so might be wary about speaking up for fear of making matters worse for themselves. For me, this fear reinforces just how vulnerable residents feel (and I know this because of how many have told me so) and how similar it seems to the emotional delicacy of women locked into abusive partnerships but who rely on that person for food and shelter.

Then there is the issue of control and that paternalistic reflex that seems to tempt so many in relations with older adults. With staff or family this can translate to a level of protection that either reduces the opportunity of an older adult to choose for themselves or engenders a culture where the older adult easily defers to others to make decisions on their behalf. Therefore, as much as not having mandatory reporting for all forms of abuse (like with children) on one level appears to be a form of complacency, on another level I appreciate that in the service of dignity, a senior deserves every morsel of control they can get their hands on – you being their "knight in shining armour" might not be representative of this.

There is also the thorny issue of capacity. Have they a sound mind or do they need specialist assessment to revise their cognitive ability status and perhaps refer to an enduring power of attorney? Maybe they need someone to appeal to an external source such as the Guardianship Board to make decisions on their behalf and protect their best interests? And finally, you have your own personal and professional ethics to consider. Are you bound by duty of care responsibilities that require you to act with due diligence – beneficence – should you learn of a situation that has compromised or might compromise the older adult's wellbeing? As well as all this you need to walk a fine line between growing trust with your client and, at the same time, with staff of the facility.

There are three things that you can do to stop you from getting stomach ulcers. First, early on in the piece when you meet with a senior, phrase any duty of care responsibilities with a positive spin toward them. For example, I might say, "If I find that you aren't well, then of course I will check that staff know about it. And if residents tell me about things that don't sound right about their care, maybe even abusive, then it makes sense to let management know because everyone has the right to feel safe and respected." It helps to try and balance an interest of protection and respect of individual choice. Second, no matter what scale of alleged misconduct or resident issue, you have behaved ethically if you remind your client of their rights. Third, when you begin working in a facility, include conversations about alleged abuse in the explanation of your role to senior staff. Agree that, where possible, you will notify them of any concerns first. This encourages trust and also sends a message that you are not going to turn a blind eye to a major transgression.

It also helps to agree that, from time to time, you may need to contact your local report line and response service[6] to sound out an issue of concern. Something to keep in mind though: even if this response service does come out to meet with a resident about alleged family abuse, they will still notice and respond to *anything* else that they do not think comes "up to scratch". This is a good thing but it can be a little uncomfortable when staff know that you are the one who instigated such a visit. This is where it really pays to have worked on your relationships with staff – built trust in your service – so that you can manage any misunderstandings that may arise from an instance like this. Ultimately, however, if a case of facility negligence emerges that just happened to be noticed as a result of your call out then addressing this takes precedence over any tension that might result between you and the facility.

The physical space

This part is really quite simple. Create opportunities for privacy and choice where you hold sessions, and choice about how that space is constructed. It is a simple concept but not as easy as you might think in its execution. Something worth keeping in mind: seniors are often deaf to some degree. This means that you need to talk quite loud at times. They also might not be very mobile, or they might be in a room shared by others. So, it pays to be prepared. Here are some pointers:

1. Know where private rooms or spaces are in each facility and how to access them.

2. See if carer staff can move the resident to their room before you introduce your service to maximize comfort. Only appear once they are in their room to avoid awkward conversations en route.

3. Have a brochure to give so, if you are only able to first meet in the public lounge area (and if they can see), they can get a quick overview of the nature of your visit and be more inclined to accept an invitation to go somewhere private so you can talk more openly (be prepared to push them yourself or get a carer to assist with a transfer).

4. If they do not seem too suspicious of you and your request to see them, ask if they do not mind you closing their door if you are alone in their room.

5. Ask if you can place a "please do not disturb" sign on their door at the second visit.

6. Know where the closest (and easy to lift) chairs are. For your own sake, do not torture yourself by sitting on a bed or a walker. And remember that commodes are not really chairs! Alternatively you could come with your own portable chair. I know of a psychotherapist in the States who does this. It is a good idea but one I have not yet implemented because I am already pulling around a travel trolley of resources.

7. Ask before moving any piece of furniture or sitting down ("Do you mind if I...?").

8. Always remember to put everything back *exactly* as you found it. The other day I was reminded about just how important

this is. The man was blind and as I was explaining that I was putting his chair back I learnt just how exact it needed to be: the correct positioning of furniture was an important part of his mobility.

9. Always (and every time) check with them how they would like you to leave their door – open, closed, half shut? Their ability to choose how they would like their door to be might be one of the few symbols of independence that they have left.

In a long-term care situation, or in any type of supported care arrangement, the infrastructure around counselling – your relationship with staff and how you navigate different situations – is vitally important. Therapeutic encounters take place in a context where many other things need to be considered. And positive outcomes are often dependent on the amount you collaborate with staff, which is what the next section is about.

Collaboration is key

Effective care of seniors cannot happen without a multi-disciplinary collaborative effort. All elements of wellbeing, which Chapter 3 will explore in more detail, interrelate with each other. More than for any other population, advanced seniors in residential facilities need the cooperation of everyone in their care team (Knight 2004), and you are a part of that team.

But while you might be an important element of this team approach to care, it is unlikely that you will be as involved as the carers, nurses, Lifestyle and other staff who interact with residents daily. They have usually forged supportive relationships with those referred to you – relationships that you can capitalize on so you can help the senior build their trust in you. Maybe have the clinical nurse introduce you if she or he thinks that reticence might be likely. Find out who someone's favourite carer is and involve them as a go-to person if the client wants you to advocate for them, or copy this person into case notes that you send to senior staff. Check in with the nurse on duty before you visit your client if they have had urinary tract infections: the extent to which it has cleared up is sure to impact on the quality (or not) of your session. Use staff knowledge to help you decide the health status of someone and, hence, how deeply you can be involved at this point in time. And certainly report any unusual changes that might signal the need for medical attention. In big ways and small, collaboration is the glue that can hold everything together (and benefit client wellbeing).

Residential care is a living, breathing organism. It can be as much the solution to senior wellbeing as it can be the problem. But there is only one way that you will be able to harness its strengths and address the challenges: understand it and breathe with it.

PERSONAL REFLECTION

1. Have you ever been in long-term care facility? What do you remember about this experience? (Who were you seeing, etc.?)

_____

_____

2. How would you describe life in long-term care?

_____

_____

3. How might these views either positively or negatively colour your future interactions in one?

_____

_____

4. What do you think might be the most challenging aspect of working as a psychotherapist in a long-term care setting?

_____

_____

5. If you were to work with seniors in hospital or long-term care settings, what opportunities do you think that you would relish the most?

_____

_____

CHAPTER 2

BARRIERS TO ENGAGEMENT

The more we understand how we can successfully engage in therapy, the better positioned we are to adopt a practice that is sensitive to client need and is relevant. This understanding, then, makes it more likely for positive therapeutic outcomes to occur. In the case of seniors it means understanding the referral context, cohort-specific issues related to attitudes and values, unfamiliarity with the concept of counselling, how much they can trust you, and how "senior friendly" you are in terms of respectful language, fitting the therapy to the person and being alert to the effects of ageism.

The referral context

As I mentioned in "A special breed of senior" in the introduction, I have found that advanced seniors in care facilities virtually never self-refer. Just as is the case with men (especially in country areas) where there can be "lower levels of help-seeking behaviours for emotional or mental health concerns compared to women" (APS 2011, topic 3, p.8), there can be different comfort levels in asking for psychological help depending on your age cohort. It often amazes me the difference with younger populations – even the "young-old" (65–74) – where they look at you as if to say, "I've got a problem, goddam it, and I want you to help me make it go away." They can easily relate to goals and what they do not want in their life anymore (notwithstanding the push-pull of differing interests). They have, to some degree, already made a commitment to the process, unless severely coerced.

Even in my role as a private practitioner under Medicare where clients have obtained a mental health care plan from their general practitioner (GP), many advanced seniors still act as though they are doing their GP or relative a favour by seeing you. They might even cleverly spin it toward being something of benefit to you, "Hopefully I can be of help to you dear." While I am often enriched by my encounters with seniors, I think you get what I mean: the session is not mine, it is theirs. The following are three possibilities as to why advanced seniors (in any context) might show wariness toward psychotherapy: cohort-specific issues for this age group whom Hugh Mackay (1997) calls "the lucky generation", being as familiar with counselling as one might be with a Martian, and complex issues around how relaxed they can actually be in baring all.

Resident unfamiliarity and wariness

Remember Harold from "A special breed of senior"? Imagine, in your first encounter, him glancing up at you suspiciously. "Who is this person, and what do they want from me?" could just as well be what he is thinking. Any "troubles" he perceives himself to have, he could just dismiss as a normal part of ageing and not see the point of investigating it further. He has not come to see you. He was not prepared for your visit (which can be a good thing because staff may not "sell" your service correctly). If you suspect that he is not sure whether to slip the chain off his internal lock and creak the door open then you would probably be right. Your "elevator speech" – or non-verbal ways – had better be good if he is to give you any time of day at all. As difficult as this stage of engagement can be (covered in more detail in Chapter 5), I love the fact that I am on trial. I think it is a wonderful act of self-appreciation that seniors often take a guarded approach to someone and something that they are not familiar with. Any trust you earn from this point on is extremely precious and well deserved in my opinion. Seeking to "prove your worth" is as much a tool as it is a deep mark of respect at the possibility of being invited in. But, as the following explores, there are many reasons why they might not want to welcome you.

The lucky generation

Well-known psychologist and social researcher, Hugh Mackay (1997), investigated three generation groups in society. His book *Generations:*

Baby Boomers, Their Parents and Their Children called those who were born around the 1920s "lucky" based on how they described themselves in a series of consultations. Mackay appreciated how their descriptor of "lucky" seemed hardly appropriate for those whose lives, "…were darkened by the twin shadows of the Great Depression and World War II" (Mackay 1997, p.14). But by their own accounts people of this generation saw themselves as having had a "charmed" existence and who have a sense of "plain enthusiasm" (pp.15 and 28 respectively) for their lot in life.

"I'm lucky," reports one senior in *Generations*, "…I was born into the peak possible time and place in history. My parents did it tough in the Depression, but that taught me some of the most important lessons of my life" (Mackay 1997, p.16). Another says, "I am grateful to my parents…for setting such strict standards" (p.23). Mackay summed up the way this generation seemed to view their life and themselves:

> The Lucky Generation are not, of course, suggesting that a depression and a war created a bed of roses for their early growth and development. On the contrary, they see themselves as having had to suffer, to sacrifice and to struggle in those early years…they believe that they have had to work hard to achieve what they have. But they also have a deep sense of gratitude at the timing of it all. (p.26)

He goes on to identify five core values that stood out from his consultations: loyalty, saving, the work ethic, the sense of mutual obligation and patriotism. I witness these values constantly in my work with older adults of the era that Mackay (1997) speaks of. I also witness an interesting mix of viewpoint: a warp and weft of experience or perception that, collectively, weave together a certain disposition. With deep gratitude, humility and concerns of being a burden, there is also unshakable pride in their resilience and a healthy stoicism to define life on their terms.

What does this mean for the psychotherapist working with them? Please, spend a moment trying to put yourself in their shoes. If you have grown up taking pride in your ability to weather adversity, do not have a strong sense of entitlement but do have a strong sense of self, do not want your frailty to define you, and have not been socialized to be comfortable sharing your feelings, how comfortable would you feel talking about changes in your mood and how motivated would you be exploring all that seems wrong with you? But we can assume, blindly, that the goods we are peddling are the best, and that lack of uptake simply means lack of interest – not questioning how we might approach things a little differently.

Think about it. At the outset, all mainstream psychological models ask that clients acknowledge an emotional or psychological problem, praise a drive to address discontentment (which can inadvertently play down values of contentment), assume a medium- to long-range view of the future, an ability to articulate goals for their wellbeing, and a blithe use of the term "wellbeing" as if all on this planet know clearly what it means.

None of the above is wrong in and of itself, it is just that it is not right for "the lucky generation". At least, certainly not at the initial stage of therapy, which Chapter 5 will explore more. What might happen if we do not consider the unique orientation of such seniors? They are likely to be very wary. Why? Because you are casting a shadow on their fortitude, you are explicitly discussing the emotional and psychological, you are focusing on limitations and not strengths, you are highlighting current need over past accomplishment, and you are adding to their sense of dependency and, possibly, guilt about being such a burden. Why would they want to tell you how bad things have been for them and think of goals for a future that could end tomorrow?

How able are we to see things from the lucky generation's point of view? Do we try? Do we question the attitudes and values that flow from the psychological models – none of which were even invented when they were young adults – that are as familiar to us as the air that we breathe? Or do we keep reassuring ourselves that our evidence base is all we need to go by? The Australian Psychological Society in their 2000 position paper on ageing called for a "paradigm shift" (p.5) grounded in principles of empowerment and recommended that "psychology move beyond a focus on deficits and problems…that psychologists contribute positively to successful ageing by supporting people in making the most of their strengths" (p.29). I agree. We could all feel luckier if we were to be "senior friendly": be consultative, step-into-their-shoes, challenge our own generational biases, and embody practices alert to ability and strengths. What could be more satisfying than transforming wariness into positive engagement?

Martians, counsellors, all the same

Have you ever tried explaining to a 93-year-old what counselling is? It is an interesting task. I encourage you to try it if you have not already. Maybe take your great-aunt aside, your grandpa or your elderly mother. Granted, they might already have a "heads up" if you are already a counsellor. Maybe you have spoken a little bit about what you do. But even so, you might find yourself scratching your head as if you are trying to explain to a new arrival with faltering English what it means to beat-around-the-bush or let-the-cat-out-of-the-bag. You might discover, with exasperation, that the only explanations that pop out of your mouth are more slang terms, only adding to the confusion! Equally, we can trip over ourselves trying to explain counselling to advanced seniors by using even more terms that they are unfamiliar with. If this does not happen to you, then I salute you, you are clearly a natural at trans-generational communication. But, if what returns to you is a slightly poker face, a polite blank stare, then you are not alone.

Knight (2004) acknowledges the need to educate seniors about therapy, and Whyte, Pachana and McKay (2012) suggest that older adults often need to be socialized into how a psychotherapist might assist them. Yes, I agree, but I would add that how and when this is done requires careful consideration. How well might they understand the language that we are using? Obviously, when you are working with clients from non-English-speaking backgrounds this task is even more challenging. In Australia, multi-cultural diversity makes it the vibrant country that it is. If you do not find yourself working in a culturally specific facility then you are sure to find many for whom English is their second language. While it is beyond the scope of this book to bridge cultural gaps in therapy, it is another layer that psychotherapists need to be alert to and be able to navigate.

For any advanced senior, no matter what cultural background, this can mean not feeling too precious about the terms that you believe describe what you do. Maybe instead of "having a therapy session," you "have a little chat" about "changes that you have noticed lately", instead of "psychological symptoms of distress"? Perhaps you can leave off the explanation about counselling until you are sure that they feel comfortable with you? You might call yourself a "counsellor" instead of a "psychotherapist" or (much worse in my opinion) a "mental health professional". They are terms that you can use if you want to establish your credibility with a doctor but if you use "mental" anything with a senior you might lose them altogether.

And why not give them an experiential understanding of counselling before any terms are used at all. "How did it feel being able to talk about these things today?" you might enquire at the end. "Well," they might answer a little sheepishly, "good." As you smile you might reply, "I'm glad, I guess that's what counselling is all about. What say we do a little bit more of that next time?" For many of us, younger than 85, we take for granted what counselling is. There might still be stigma in the community, but at least there is (more or less) understanding. Exploring it with a senior can be like watching a child, wide-eyed with wonder and wariness, at a big new world that they are learning about for the very first time. Gradually, little by little, trust and respect are formed. For those of you well versed in the importance of a therapeutic alliance you will know that, for any population, trust is not an optional extra. It is the bedrock of any future work, and can even be therapeutic in and of itself.

Can they trust you (really)?

As just mentioned, I believe that there is nothing more important than trust. It can be what allows a client to take off their mask and bare their soul. It is something that I never take for granted. I am in constant awe at the leap of faith many take in the counselling relationship as they tell you things that they have not admitted even to themselves. It truly is quite humbling. And if developing trust is important for the general population of clients we see, then it is even more important for seniors – especially those who are intimately cared for by others.

You have been seeing Mrs Grim for six sessions now. Her willingness to engage in psychotherapy was tentative at first – it took three sessions before she agreed to be part of more formal or explicit intervention. But she now seems to warm to your presence and she is beginning to share with you her feelings about living in a residential care facility. She is always quick to point out to you the many things that she appreciates, but you suspect that there is more to her story and begin to encourage her to share. When she sighs and looks at you tentatively before saying, "Oh, but, listen to me! Silly isn't it?"

you gently remind her of the counsellor's role, how there is no "right or wrong" in what she feels, and how helpful it can be to talk things through with a professional. This seems to reassure her and she begins to be even more candid about her experiences.

At your first formal session you give her the option of just informing senior staff that you have visited (for their records) or giving them your case note each time (that her GP gets also). You explain the pros and cons and she asks if you could decide for her. After getting distracted by being asked for her meal preference – something which appears very important to her – she offhandedly answers your question finally by choosing that her notes also be forwarded to facility staff. At the seventh session, her bottom lip begins to tremble. When you ask her what the matter is – is it something that she would like to talk about – she bursts into tears.

Now imagine, if you will, a few different scenarios that could emerge as you strengthen your therapeutic alliance with Mrs Grim:

1. She tells you of an experience of incest, something that she has kept a secret for eight decades but that has been eating away at her all this time – her move to this facility only worsening experiences of shame and self-doubt. You write in your notes, that facility staff also get, "Upset about an experience of incest at the hands of her father" instead of "Upset over an incident that happened years ago". Josie, an enrolled nurse, able to administer medicines better than she can tact, blurts out the next day, "Mrs Grim! I am so sorry to hear about how your father abused you! That's just dreadful! You poor thing! Honestly, I don't know how people like that live with themselves." You get a message that Mrs Grim no longer wants to continue with therapy.

2. She tells you how she wishes she was not here. How everyone is so busy and she feels like just a number. She explains that she appreciates the care that she

receives but that no one seems to really acknowledge her as a person (except you). You write in your notes, "Upset because she feels ignored and invisible at the facility" instead of "Upset over some experiences related to facility living". Miranda, the registered nurse, is horrified. She worries that her staff have not been doing their job properly. Seeking to right a wrong she trots over to Mrs Grim's room. "Mrs Grim! I've just seen the counsellor's notes. Who is it? Who is ignoring you? You know that we love to have you here! You're our favourite Mrs G!" You get a message that Mrs Grim no longer wants to continue with therapy.

3. She tells you how desperate she is to be independent. She confesses to you that she does not use her walker to get around her room like she knows she is supposed to. She explains that she has suffered so much loss that she could not bear to lose her ability to make this one small decision for herself. You explain your concern but she answers, "Risk! I'm 88! Do you think I don't know about consequences? If I fall, I fall. I won't like it, but at least I have done things my own way." You write in your notes, "Upset because of how much independence she has lost. Gets around it by deciding not to use her walker in her room" instead of "A number of issues related to independence discussed today". She is chastised by anxious staff to use her walker. "At all times!" they implore to her. She is embarrassed and enraged and sends a message to discontinue therapy.

Grim indeed. Perhaps I am being a little extreme, but I wonder if the way we manage privacy and empowerment in therapy with seniors should be like the lengths we take to ensure safety with people experiencing domestic violence. We might check first with how they would like this session written up, check that if we give a woman any handout that her abusive partner cannot find it, that if we call, where might we say we are from, etc. These precautions are to ensure that you do not unwittingly make matters worse for your client. The same precautions could be said to be valid in work with seniors. For example, it can pay to double check or regularly check if your client would prefer the full casenote sent to care staff or, for privacy reasons so long as it does not conflict with duty of care, to simply forward the date that you saw them. And if you write something down on a card for your client – perhaps a list to honour frustrations experienced that include family – how might it look if their daughter finds it? Yes, you guessed it: learnt that one the hard way.

Positive psychology?

It is heartening indeed that at the turn of the 21st century, the field of positive psychology began to gather momentum. Now we have the International Positive Psychology Association (IPPA), championed largely by Martin Seligman who is the senior advisor of IPPA, which has as its focal point not pathology but what enables individuals and communities to thrive (IPPA 2017).

Thankfully, this scientific field of study has also spilled over into theory, research and practice with seniors. How can we view seniors more positively and what conditions make it more likely for a senior to live a happier life rich with meaning, a desirable achievement in developmental theory (APS 2000)? They are exciting new frameworks with which to view ageing. For example, the contextual, cohort-based, maturity, specific-challenge model (CCMSC) has been developed which seeks to view adult development in more positive terms than the more traditional loss-deficit model of ageing (Knight 2004). To give an example of each dimension, a context could be long-term care, a cohort effect might be the social-historical life experience related to a particular age group, an element of maturity could involve aspects like cognitive complexity or multiple family experiences, and specific challenge could refer to chronic illness or grief (Knight 2004, p.6) The CCMSC model represents an interest in moving away from unhelpful stereotypes. Similarly, phrases coming out of the positive psychology movement like "successful ageing", "healthy ageing", "positive ageing" are all catchphrases that represent attitudes and practices filled with respect and optimism (APS 2000), all of which are implicit in the 21 internationally recognized guidelines for psychological practice with older adults (APA 2014) mentioned in the introduction.

Another example of this more positive slant is Robert Hill's (2008) book *Seven Strategies for Positive Aging* that aims to assist older adults make the most out of their circumstances:

- You can find meaning in old age.

- You're never too old to learn.

- You can use the past to cultivate wisdom.

- You can strengthen life-span relationships.

- You can promote growth through giving and receiving help.

- You can forgive yourself and others.

- You can possess a grateful attitude.

(p.xii)

The developments of positive psychology and positive ageing are, in my opinion, very welcome. They challenge disempowering and disrespectful conceptions of inability and a generalized view of ageing that leave no room for notions of vitality, wisdom and fulfilment no room for strengths and possibilities. So it is intriguing to me, or perhaps understandable given the youth of positive psychology, that language and orientation in relation to seniors still seem laced with disempowering concepts related to pathology – and this by practitioners who I believe have a very deep and real commitment to the wellbeing of older adults.

Let me ask you something, would you like to be associated with the term "geriatric"? No? Why is that? Perhaps some things come to mind like "lost cause" or "loopy". Yes, geriatric is a medical term that has its roots in science but, on the street, it is not as neutral. So what about looking more closely at language as it relates to seniors? From a Narrative Therapy standpoint, "When engaging in language, we are not engaging in a neutral activity...our understandings of our lived experience, including those that we refer to as 'self-understandings', are mediated through language" (White and Epston 1989, p.31). Therefore if the word "geriatric" has negative connotations in everyday language then why do we use it – even in a peer to peer discussion about older adult affairs? Could using it potentially interfere with a clinician's attitude toward those in their care or erode a senior's self-esteem?

Why not have the "Senior's Depression Scale" instead of the "Geriatric Depression Scale" because how would you feel if, through implication, it sounded like you were a geriatric with depression? Might you feel a little depressed? Even if the word "geriatric" is not said out loud it still puzzles me why this word is used so freely in psychology contexts for older adults.

And what about literature that appears to have a positive ageing bent but has phrases like "behavioural deficits", "failed to progress", "disorders" and implores practitioners to make decisions about what type of "psychological problem" the client has? This is, no doubt, a contentious area and one argument could be: If you do not know what is wrong then how can you treat it? But what if, in our interests to scrutinize every element of a senior's being through the lens of medicine, we inadvertently create more psychological problems than we solve?

Mainstream psychological practice can place with it too much focus on diagnosis: forming an understanding of the senior through a loss-deficit model. Consider the following quote:

> To form a clear picture of an older client, all elderly clients seen *must* be asked about their medical status, chronic diseases, and current acute diseases. (emphasis mine, Knight 2004, p.101)

Must? I have not found that it is imperative for me to know, let alone ask, a senior their list of ailments in order for effective therapy to occur. I understand the useful nature of a medical investigation if aspects of ability and suitability for therapy are unclear but this can be gained through consultation with staff. I am interested primarily in how the client views their situation – what problems they see as the issue. I can determine what I need to through observation, clarification and forming a person-centred approach to learning about what is important to them. Why should we encourage a self-definition around illness by impressing on the senior a need to articulate all that is "wrong" with them?

Proponents of Solution Focused Therapy – a meta model favouring a focus on client strengths – similarly observe the widespread use and limitations of problem-focused approaches that are akin to deficit models. For example, Bodmer Lutz (2014, p.5) notes that, "In traditional problem-focussed therapy, the clinician serves as expert and a thorough understanding of the problem and symptoms is necessary before treatment begins." This area is sure to be one where people have differing views, but it is my opinion that it is neither useful nor respectful to kick contact off with a focus on pathology.

Psychological institutions themselves warn against "pathologising of older persons' experiences" (APS 2000, p.3). It is too easy in our medically saturated therapeutic models to fuse the person with the problem. The Australian Psychological Society add that, "the language we choose does matter" (APS 2000, p.32). I agree, and my thoughts go back to the quote I mentioned earlier by the founders of Narrative Therapy on never assuming that language is neutral. We need to be alert to how language can keep people locked into negative "truths" about their identity, robbing them from empowering self-definitions, and seek opportunities for alternative story development and more liberating conceptions of self. Ignoring opportunities to examine how potentially disempowering certain labels or phrases are, I believe, is a form of maleficence.

When we speak in terms of abnormality or disorders, how are seniors likely to feel? Might their situation be more a case of being "abnormal for them" rather than "evidence of abnormality" which locates abnormality internally to them instead of externally? How might we feel if we have lost all we held dear with no chance of escape? Not quite like our normal self? And if our low mood seems to be a sign that we have not adjusted – developed an adjustment disorder – what exactly are we expected to adjust to or accept? An erasing of any semblance of our former self as we also kiss goodbye what used to be a feisty spirit? I suggest that what is more disordered is how some can view the experience of life transition. Yes, integration and a level of acceptance can eventually ease distress but the older adult is not disordered if their life has become unrecognizable. In the words of Michael White, founder of Narrative Therapy, "The person is never the problem; the problem is the problem" (Sween 1998, p.4).

Finally, quests to empower older adults to embrace a more optimistic mindset can open up the possibility for a more meaningful (and ultimately happier) life. But I believe that this interest to be positive needs to be tempered with a watchful eye for when seniors feel more ensnared by the mantra of positivity than empowered by it, more burdened by an expectation to be happy than an allowing for the unpleasant. Could we, by encouraging with such vigour the importance of a bright outlook, unwittingly make it even more difficult for seniors to face change and loss with dignity?

Too many times I have witnessed a senior racked with self-recrimination that they are not being positive enough. Perhaps "the lucky generation" do not need a focus on resilience and positivity as much as younger generations? They have already chalked up a lifetime of points in being able to face the world bravely. Maybe the time for them now is to look at themselves and their situation in a softer light? The tenets of Acceptance and Commitment Therapy could be relevant here in an interest to offset any fallout in the pursuit of happiness and positivity: better to observe and "sit with" unpleasant thoughts and emotions than get caught up in a struggle trying to be free of them (Harris 2007, 2009).

If psychotherapists working with older adults truly want to embrace "positive psychology", then perhaps their language could be a bit more, um, positive. And while the ideal of being positive is admirable, perhaps we can also remind seniors that not feeling positive is not negative. It just *is*. When we stop to consult seniors about how they view the world, learn about a particular generational orientation, then we are in a better position to create therapy contexts that are relaxed, engaging and productive. Being alert to the possible conditions behind resident wariness can help you turn potentially awkward encounters into fruitful ones. Being prepared to explain your role and the counselling process *in a way that seniors understand and feel comfortable with* is one step toward this goal. Another is to ensure that you develop a relationship and adhere to protocols which centre around the promotion of trust.

Other avenues that can reduce feelings of alienation, disempowerment or wariness for seniors include a reflective monitoring of what words you use to describe older adults and your work with them. While this communication may not always be directly with them, ensuring a respectful orientation can only be of benefit. In Chapter 8 we will also consider how ageist attitudes in our society can further complicate successful engagement. Finally, positive ageing practices offer an important framework on how to view older adults generally, and how to engage with them specifically. However, a focus on the positive needs to be tempered with an understanding of how encouraging it with too much vigour can lead people to feel less than positive about themselves, failures even. By all means encourage a positive outlook, so long as by doing so it does not make it negative.

PERSONAL REFLECTION

1. What aspects of "the lucky generation" were you not aware of?

_____

_____

2. Is this new knowledge likely to change the way you interact with seniors in the future? If so, how?

_____

_____

3. What was the most thought-provoking section for you in this chapter?

_____

_____

4. What do you think about the notion that elements of mainstream psychology might be disempowering for seniors?

_____

_____

5. What ways have you tried to put clients or seniors at ease in the past? What does this say about your attributes and values?

_____

_____

CHAPTER 3

TYPES OF DISTRESS

Understanding the types of distress common, but not inevitable, for advanced seniors can give you an ability to better empathize: both emotionally and practically. As a psychotherapist you would be no stranger to the idea of empathizing with your clients. We use our skills of intuition and emotional engagement to develop a productive therapeutic bond. In the case of seniors, it can be advantageous to also foster practical empathy: developing a therapeutic alliance by being attuned to practical issues which might increase client comfort and engagement. If you have spent any time working in the disability or palliative care sector then this notion will be familiar to you.

For example, if someone is not able to stand then you direct all contact to them while sitting, instead of talking down to them. If you are visiting someone in a hospital bed then you might ensure that your position in the room is one which minimizes strain to their neck. If you are seeing a homeless person then you might consider how helpful it could be that they have some food in their belly before you begin. A person with a speech impediment might appreciate being able to write their thoughts down, and so on. Therefore, the following hopes to highlight common forms of distress for seniors with the view to develop a comprehensive empathetic stance. In this way, not only are you learning to see things from their point of view, thereby "walking" with them more closely, but you are also considering how you can make counselling more accessible and comfortable for that person. To take this journey, I invite you now to recall Harold, as his story will help us explore the types of distress common to the advanced senior.

Physical

The yellow hospital blanket sinks conspicuously down on one side of Harold's body. "That's all I got now," he says glancing at his lower limbs. You are not sure whether to follow his line of sight or stay looking at him, so you settle for trying to take in the whole story. He tries to move his left leg then winces, his face crunches tight. "Even this one gives me stick." Then he looks at you and adds through still gritted teeth, "Peripheral arterial disease – PAD – means my blood doesn't flow so well. It's part of the diabetes." You admire out loud his ability to say the full medical term, and suggest that it could be tricky to say if you were drunk. A chuckle bubbles up and his chest wobbles for a bit. Your gaze returns to the contemplative and it appears that this waft of humour has been appropriate and helpful.

Harold volunteers more of his story, his voice gaining strength. While the amputation is the most obvious physical change for Harold, like peeling an onion, you learn of other layers: excruciating pain, sleeplessness, infections and increased medication resulting in side effects. There are also other physical changes, not all related to diabetes: reduced hearing in his left ear (you have observed this and moved your seat to his good ear), diminished eye sight, "gammy" hands and bed sores that require painful turning. "It's not the same body I used to have," Harold says, his eyes a mixture of pain and reminiscence, but softer toward you than when you first arrived.

For many advanced seniors, the list of physical change and decline can be like the rolling credits of a Star Wars movie and pain is the monster that everyone is trying to shoo away. There are of course medication and other strategies for management (discussed in Chapter 6), but living with persistent pain can be a fly-in-the-ointment experience of ageing.

Another physical issue that can cause considerable distress – but can (literally) be a silent issue – is deafness. Whether in the community or in a facility, the experience of deafness can limit opportunities for social nourishing. Even with the aid of a hearing device deafness can frustrate and isolate. Ringing or reverberations in the ear can be a constant irritation – the extent difficult to explain to others – and when deafness is acquired late in life there is a good chance that reduced sight will make lip reading difficult also.

Engaging in therapeutic relations with someone who is deaf can be tricky too. It is not so comfortable yelling at the top of your lungs a sensitive reflection, "So you feel really sad and lonely at the moment?" And trying to deliver a soothing guided meditation is out of the question. One therapist I know of uses a laptop to type questions or comments for her clients which I think is a very clever remedy but there are still bound to be frustrations on both sides when trying to offer counselling to someone with a hearing impairment.

Some are bothered more than others by their physical ailments, but the experience of physical decline – and the physical world – is as familiar to seniors as meteorological readings are to a pilot. It is just something that has to be navigated. Like a Dalmatian, their days are dotted by tablet regimes, doctor appointments, supported care schedules and physio treatment. All a reminder of what no longer is.

Sometimes a focus on improving the physical can give a sense of purpose – for everyone – keeping at bay the ugly truth that things are winding down. "I'm gonna get these legs walking better though!" they might say, with the intensity befitting an Olympic athlete. And sometimes that same determination can be a masking of grief. Criticisms about how staff are not doing enough to help them reach their goals may really be about how they are starting to see the "writing on the wall", an indirect protest against their failing body.

Neurological

At your second session the way Harold greets you reminds you of many other residents. It is as if he is thinking, "I know I've met this person before but I'd be damned if I knew what it was about. Bloody memory! I feel like such a fool." Sensing that he is trying to match your air of purpose with as much of-course-I-know-who-you-are pretence as possible, you spare him the indignity of guessing details and simply state your name, your role and a brief synopsis of your last meeting. Later, you suggest to him that many people in his age bracket notice changes to memory – is this the case for him? "Well, I don't think I'm going bloody senile if that's what you mean!" he replies somewhat offended. You admit that this can be a fear of most, but also that there can be many reasons for memory loss. With the amount of pain and sleeplessness he is enduring, actually absorbing information might be a bigger barrier for him right now than retrieval.

Gently, you inquire some more and you acknowledge how distressing memory issues – whether it be transient or degenerative – can be, another loss. You explore with him a memory support tool that you can use in therapy to increase confidence. It is a simple solution, you explain. "I'll just bring an exercise book with me next time. I'll write in there a summary of each session, things that have stood out for you as being important. You can use it to review what we've said, practise anything that might be relevant, remind yourself of the date and time of next session, and write in it like a journal if you want to or are able. Elizabeth can also communicate to me through it if she wants and if it's okay with you." He now appears more settled and you wonder if it is because your inquiry about his memory issues did not turn into a neon sign of "deficit" for him.

Memory issues, like the sort Harold is having, is just one example of why a senior might experience neurological-related distress. Your resident may be in the early or middle stages of dementia (diagnosed or not) as Harold could be. Knight (2004) has provided an excellent reference for psychotherapy in this context through his chapter, "The Person With Dementia". Hence, there is no need to duplicate anything here, but I would like to share with you a quote of his that I particularly like:

> It is undeniable that changes occur in the brains of persons with dementia. The changes are gradual over a period of years, however, and although important functions and aspects of the person are lost during that time, they are not lost all at once. The assumption that new learning is impossible is likewise an oversimplification and an instance of the fallacy of all-or-none thinking. Is new learning more

difficult for persons with dementia? Of course it is. It is impossible? Not until the latest stages of the disease. (Knight 2004, p.187)

Probably about 60 per cent of my clientele at any given time are at some stage of dementia, and yet therapy often concludes with an appraisal – from them and me – that our sessions have eased distress. It is not true, in my opinion, that you "cannot teach an old dog new tricks". While neurological changes in the form of dementia can present their challenges, psychotherapy is still a viable option. On this point, I also appreciate the clarification that Knight (2004) provides:

> It would be wrong to deprive persons in the early stages of dementia of the benefits of appropriate psychological intervention. It would also be wrong (fraudulent) to provide verbally based, insight-orientated therapy to nonverbal persons in the late stages of dementia. (p.190)

Before we finish with dementia, however, I would like to mention the incidence of language reversion. In their autumn issue, the *Journal of the Australian Association of Social Workers* included a paper entitled, "Language reversion among people with dementia from culturally and linguistically diverse backgrounds: the family experience" (Tipping and Whiteside 2015).

The incidence that the authors spoke of reminded me of a Dutch lady I once saw. She had been a resident of Australia for decades, spoke English well, but had begun to interlace her conversation with her language of birth as she progressed with dementia. Mostly, she was unaware of the sliding nature of her bilingual expression. She relied on her daughter to encourage conversion back to English and, especially, to translate when this was not possible.

While my client was obviously not comfortable with her daughter knowing the intimate details of her distress – she did not want to burden her – she equally knew that this was the only context in which our sessions could take place and decided that the benefit was worth the cost. In this time I was particularly struck with how much we rely on non-verbal language to communicate. When this lady was speaking in Dutch it surprised me how much I could understand her emotional position based on her facial expressions and helped me appreciate how useful these observations can be with seniors – or anyone – when language presents as a barrier.

Other degenerative neurological conditions that you are likely to come across in a long-term care setting are illnesses like multiple sclerosis (MS), Parkinson's and Huntington's disease. My years as the social worker/counsellor for people with MS often took me to long-term care facilities and if you are referred people with such a condition you are likely to find that they are significantly younger than the usual "crowd" in a facility – an understandable bone of contention.

Technically not degenerative, but still likely to be accumulative, is distress related to a stroke or transient ischaemic attacks (TIAs) – often called "mini strokes". In the case of TIAs, while an entire half of someone's body may not be affected as in the case of a stroke, the presentation can be very complex if multiple TIAs continue – minor but very diffuse damage to the brain usually described as vascular dementia. In these instances assessing through the Mini Mental State Examination[7] can help to ascertain what level of functioning is present so you can either modify therapy accordingly or decide that this client is unsuitable for your service.

As mentioned before, our observation of the non-verbal can be an important tool in helping us understand our client. This is no truer than when there is a significant speech impediment due to neurological degeneration or impact (or in the case of a physical issue like pulmonary heart disease – insufficient oxygen). In times like these speech can be incredibly laboured and sometimes you need to sit on your hands and count to ten (or 20!) before opening your mouth. Yes, you might have awkward moments like the time delay in a Skype chat, but with patience you can begin to look out for subtle signs that tell you when your client still has more to say. It may be a little twitch of the mouth, a slight breath in, or glance toward you. This is where expectations of therapeutic goals can sort of go tumbling down the hill and you are left with trying, as best you can, to simply be present and create space for expression.

Social or spiritual

There is a pause in your conversation and something takes your eye: medals in a frame on the wall, blue ribbons and a picture. You ask Harold if you can take a closer look and admire his collection of prize-winning achievements. His voice is still heavy with depression but there is a change that you notice in his tone. Pride begins to lightly touch each word and each recollection of his days spent playing lawn bowls or being a volunteer groundsman.

He also speaks of his mates Colin, Ralph, Chuck and Des who also used to enjoy watching football with him. Colin, you hear, has got Alzheimer's and Ralph is the only one he has contact with now. You discover how Ralph visits Harold weekly, how he has urged Harold to come to the club but at this point he implores to you, "Look at me! How could I see them like this?" It is a rhetorical question, you choose not to accept the invitation of an answer, but shelve the push-pull nature of his social needs for another time – once trust has developed a little more.

There are other pictures around, on the walls and ledges. Conversation turns to family and his wife Elizabeth. "I miss her," he says simply and his bottom lip begins to tremble, "we used to do so much together, and now –". Harold tries to shield his face away from you and then admonishes himself, "Crying like a baby, aren't I?" You stay a silent compassionate witness to his pain, and he continues telling you about his beloved whom he can no longer be with in the same way as before. Your mind wafts to your own loved ones and your stomach tugs in recognition of his loss – of the basic human need for connection and belonging.

In under a year Harold's life has been turned upside down, done a complete 360 degrees. He has gone from being independent, capable, highly involved in his local bowling club and living at home with his wife, to 24/7 nursing care and detached from his community. The web of social losses can be many for advanced seniors in long-term care. Often their pathway into care looks a lot like a rather sinister life version of the game of Monopoly. Instead of "go directly to jail, do not pass go, do not collect 200 dollars", it is "go directly to facility living, do not go home, do not go back to life as you knew it". The shock related to this abrupt flushing of all-that-felt-right-and-good can be very much akin to an experience of trauma.

I should reiterate, at this point, that not all to whom this pathway relates experience distress, not all who live in a facility context feel disconnected (some indeed flourish with new found relationships), and not all who live in the community feel isolated or grief stricken by the death of a husband or wife (some are glad to finally be free of them!). For example, studies have shown that psychological wellbeing in old age generally paints a positive picture (APS 2000, p.17). The point is, however, that to work effectively with seniors demands a sensitivity to all the different ways in which people can experience distress. The tenets of the CCMSC model – contextual, cohort-based, maturity, specific challenge – are relevant here in that acknowledgement is given to the *individual* and their own *unique* set of circumstances that may be radically different from another person's of similar age or other type of grouping.

In relation to spiritual distress, I am reminded of an indigenous woman who I once saw. Not only was she grieving the recent loss of a relative, which triggered the loss of a long deceased son, but she was a recent admission to the facility and a long way from her "mob". As much as she felt cared for by facility staff, she felt uncomfortable wailing in the way that she would normally if she were amongst other indigenous women engaged in traditional healing. She was not able to attend the funeral (held a very long way away) and there were complex reasons that prevented her from being effectively supported by her family who lived locally. Being acutely aware of my ignorance, I explored with her other culturally appropriate ways for her to grieve. Mainly this involved a rudimentary version of "clapping sticks" where she sang in her own language and shed many tears. She said this helped her "Be the song, and bring the song back." For this woman, it was not only a social disconnection that had caused her distress (on top of grief), but a cultural and spiritual one too.

A sense of disconnection can be a persistent problem for seniors. Solutions that younger generations employ to reduce distance – phoning, email, social media – do not work so well if you are deaf, computer illiterate or scared (or both), have vision impairment, uncooperative hands or limited resources (financial and human) to help you overcome barriers to communication. If you are living in a facility you may have a limited pool of like-minded, cognitively intact residents who are also able to hear what you are saying. Since moving into a facility you might have also developed a longer list of people-I-want-to-avoid. And even when enjoyable relationships are formed with fellow residents or kind carers, there is a high chance that this will soon be lost due to death or staff turnover. True, I mainly listen to those for whom life is not so great, but many tell me of how lonely they feel and how they long for deeply satisfying connection with others (bingo might not float their boat).

Psychological

Harold looks down at his hands for a moment. "Yes," he quietly offers. You acknowledge, by way of giving him the breather that he seems to need, that these are pretty tough questions. "Is it okay to continue?" Yes. You look at question number 12 from the Geriatric Depression Scale Long Form, "Do you prefer to stay in your room, rather than going out and doing new things?" Yes. "Do you frequently worry about the future?" Yes. "Do you feel you have more problems with memory than most?" Yes. "Do you think it is wonderful to be alive now?" N- . Harold's response is interrupted by a knock at the door, followed by nurse Nancy bursting in despite your "therapy in progress" sign. "Sorry love, but this is important." You turn as her rattling trolley sidles up near you and wonder quietly to yourself, and this isn't? "So!" nurse Nancy says brightly to Harold as she hands him his tablets. "How are you going today? Good?" Harold smiles graciously, and nurse Nancy turns on her heels to finish the rest of her tight routine. The mood feels more awkward as you return to your questions and you work hard to bring Harold back to a sense of ease. The questionnaire is now complete and your pen dances down the page doing the math: 27 out of 30, in the range of "severe depression". You sensitively share these results with Harold and explain the importance of alerting his medical practitioner.

As discussed in the introduction, the findings from the Depression in Residential Aged Care study (Commonwealth of Australia 2013), where 52 per cent of residents had clinical indications of depression, is likely to be an underestimation. In addition, depression in older adults comes with a number of risk factors:

Risk factors for the development of depression include: female gender, social isolation, widowhood, physical ill health, disability, chronic pain, recent bereavement, a family history of depression, and a past history of depression. Prevalence rates of depression in cases of stroke, Parkinson's disease, disability, and dementia range upward from 20% (Snowdon 1997). If untreated, depression is likely to persist and is a predictor of premature death (see review by Zisook and Downs 1998). One consequence of depression can be suicide. The three main risk factors for suicide in older people are: depression, social isolation, and chronic pain. (APS 2000, p.19)

Examples of suicide among older adults are many. Much loved Australian author Nikki Gemmel (2017) describes the devastation of losing her elderly mother, who was in persistent pain,[8] to suicide in her book *After*. I am also remembering that, just in this last fortnight, I have seen two women in care facilities who had strong intentions to end their life after experiencing a significant number of changes and loss. The American Psychological Association report on their website that "Older adults have the highest rates of suicide of any age group, and this is particularly pronounced among men" (Scogin 2009). Furthermore, the American Association for Marriage and Family Therapy reveal on their website that:

> In 2002, the annual suicide rate for persons over the age of 65 was over 15 per 100,000 individuals; this number increases for those aged 75 to 84, with over 17 suicide deaths per every 100,000. The number rises even higher for those over age 85. Further, elder suicide may be under-reported by 40% or more. (American Association for Marriage and Family Therapy 2017)

The experience of psychological distress for older adults, in facility or community living, is real and very sobering. Dysphoria may be a niggling sense that things are no longer the same or, like in Harold's case, it could be extreme. It might be a clear-cut presentation of depression, grief or anxiety, or a combination of many things. Seniors may be more comfortable locating the problem as something physical – "I'm just so tired lately, but you know, I guess that's what you expect at my age" – and be reluctant or unable to express their problem in terms of mood (Bogenburger 2014; Whyte, Pachana and McKay 2012). Or sometimes a fixation on food quality is really just code for "I'm not coping." Your language, again, might be important to consider. For example, I find that advanced seniors relate more readily to "feeling tense and worried a lot" versus having anxiety; "sad a lot of the time" rather than depressed; "frustrated" or "irritated" instead of angry – especially for women.

For many, psychological distress appears intimately related to perceptions of self. Can they still see themselves as active if they can no longer walk? Can they see themselves as hospitable if they can no longer cook? Can they see themselves as competent if they are thrown by this thing called age? The many changes that can occur, especially sudden moves into facility living or marked deterioration in ability, can make it challenging for seniors to hold onto a core identity and feel good about themselves. In these instances, psychotherapists can play a strong role in the assessment and treatment for distress so that quality of life (and an interest in it) is entertained as much as is possible.

Environmental or lifestyle

Arthur, Harold's room mate, is being wheeled out just as you enter his room for your session. "Blurghhh! Urgh, urgh, blurghh!" A cacophony of coughing follows Arthur all the way down the corridor. "Poor bugger," Harold says. "Pneumonia. Coughs like that for most of the night." It is your fourth session now with Harold and you are getting a clearer picture about how difficult it is for him to get a good night's sleep – between his pain and Arthur's coughing – which no doubt also affects mood and memory. His doctor and nurses know about this, however, and are trying to manage as best they can with medication. Harold, you learn, has requested a single room but is in the queue with many others. You suggest trying earplugs and he asks you to write that down in the communication book for his wife. "At least," Harold points out, "they take him out for most of the day."

There are other noises that Harold has to listen to: in one session you hear a blood-curdling cry. Harold second guesses your startled expression. "It's all right, it happens all the time. I think she's, you know, poor love –." Alzheimer's is noted if not spoken of. Yes, with "ageing in place" you are well aware of the eclectic mix you can have in any cluster of rooms, and how full dementia wards usually are. "Another noise to put up with, eh?" you enquire. It is more a validation than a question and Harold nods his head seeming to appreciate this acknowledgement.

If you have ever felt slightly nauseous walking through an aged care facility, puckered your face against a smell, observed a grown woman clutching a dolly with desperation, felt a flood of melancholy as death fills your view – then you are in a perfect position to be a supportive psychotherapist for those whose lives are peppered with this every day.

For people like Harold, environmental distress can mean anything from noisy neighbours, to being constantly confronted by death and decline, to dealing with a shortage of staff when you are busting to go. Lifestyle losses and changes can include an increased reliance on others for personal care, a radically shrunk diet of satisfying recreational options, and having to have dinner at a time when children usually do. It is not that there can be no joy in facility living, it is just that sometimes it is not enjoyable. Some of these losses can be addressed; others not so easily. However, I would like to offer an example here of how simple policy or advocacy measures could make the world of difference for some seniors.

One 95-year-old client comes to mind. She had been told upon admission to the facility that none of the residents were allowed the code to leave the building – that if she were to exit the building she would need to do so only with a staff member or family assisting her. When I first met with this intelligent, resilient and resourceful woman – she spent decades managing her family's home and farming estate in a remote region of Australia after her husband died – the words that seared through my heart were "I feel like I'm in jail. I have no option of escape." A few sessions later, immediately after her 95th birthday, she told me again of how it tortures her to not have freedom to step out of the facility's walls, "What's my crime? To have lived as long as I have?" She looked indignant, and this level of restriction certainly appeared to me to be unjustified. She was cognisant, responsible and got around ably on her walker. Why could she not just step outside of her own volition and smell the outside air? In fact this resident said that even if she were not allowed to leave without assistance – just knowing that she *could* would significantly improve her appraisal of facility living. She also felt shame for feeling this way. Her family's response to her distress was, she told me with a painful look, "But mum, you have everything you need!"

With the client's permission (albeit reluctantly because she was afraid to be seen as a trouble maker) I posed this question to the clinical nurse. The nurse agreed with me about her cognitive ability and responsible nature but looked worried – what if she fell? I explained the psychological impact of not being trusted and she got my point. She stressed that as long as the resident understood the need for her to be supervised if she went beyond a couple of steps then she could get the access. My client was elated. She could feel free – think it even if she decided to not act on it under the conditions specified. But despite this achievement, what worried me was how much of this distress was avoidable if different admission policies were in place – ones that did not have a blanket "thou shalt never be free again!" ring to them. And the more sobering question for me was: how many other older people in care are there globally who feel just like her – unjustifiably jailed. For life. Just because they still live.

As the above case illustrates, distress can overlap. The example above related to psychological distress born out of environmental or lifestyle issues. Therefore types of distress, as seen in Figure 3.1, can be seen as an evolving and fluctuating group of issues that often feed into the other. If you had a major stroke (neurological) then you might have ended up living in a facility which significantly changed your circumstances (environmental or lifestyle), brought on by multiple limitations (physical), affecting your ability to socialize (social), which has resulted in depressive presentations (psychological). Similarly, challenges for an older adult fulfilling sexual health needs might be a cause-and-effect mix of the environmental where there is reduced privacy, the physical, social – especially if stigma surrounds an alternative orientation – and the psychological where identity and self-esteem issues are relevant. Successful ageing is about using therapy to understand these interdependent elements and optimize wellbeing in as many areas as is possible.

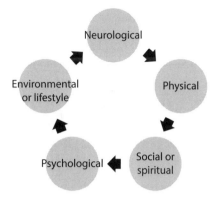

Figure 3.1: Types of resident distress

Professor Nancy Pachana (2016) adds to this understanding of cause and effect by discussing the dimensions of primary and secondary ageing. For example, in relation to physical or biological issues "muscle mass and bone density decline" can begin as a primary change but become "disability as a result of injury" which is a secondary change (p.23). Therefore senior distress can be related to the interaction between types of wellbeing *and* also related to the change or decline *within* each type, creating a complex web of secondary or even tertiary issues. In the next chapter we will also look at dynamic processes: the moving wheel of assessment.

PERSONAL REFLECTION

1. What parts of Harold's story in this chapter were most confronting?

_____

_____

2. Was there a type of distress you had not considered? If so, which one was it?

_____

_____

3. Which type of distress would you feel most comfortable working with?

_____

_____

4. Which type of distress would you feel least comfortable talking about?

_____

_____

5. How do you feel so far about Harold and his situation?

_____

_____

— PART 2 —

INTERVENTION

CHAPTER 4

THE MOVING WHEEL OF ASSESSMENT

Just as distress can be an evolving mix of circumstance – a fluid presentation of need – so too can the task of assessing and addressing it be like a wheel in constant motion. Psychotherapists are surveyors of the human soul. We are ever aware of the microscopic and the grand as our clients reveal themselves to us. Depending on our training, what we notice and how we interact with that information varies, but there is one goal that yokes us together – a desire to understand and relieve people of their problems. Your powers of observation and your ability to pick your way through situations of delicate complexity are probably what moved you toward psychotherapy in the first place. And all the while, whether formally or informally, you assess so you can judge where you might place your next step.

Your desire to empower clients and bring about constructive change is as relevant for older adults as it is for any other population. But here is the thing: not only do you need to discern what the key issue appears to be, but also whose problem it is, whether this problem is something your service can address, and how you might go about respectfully working with (a mostly unsuspecting) older adult to get a clearer picture of need. Yes, responding to residential or community referrals for older adults and successfully determining the core issue can be a little like working your way through dense jungle. But I can promise you one thing, you are not likely to be bored! Guidance can be helpful. So, the following discussion hopes to build in you an understanding of the mental health and neurological spectrum, confidence in determining suitability, and skills in getting to the heart of the matter. So, instead of feeling overwhelmed, you can breathe deeply in and see clearly the path before you.

The mental health and neurological spectrum

The nurse's eyes are wide as she tells you about their latest admission. "Moved in four days ago she did. A friend of hers brought her in; was her neighbour I think. Said it took some convincing, Mrs Constance put up a bit of a fight, but she's known this friend a while and eventually agreed to come and live here. The friend looked exhausted. Now I can understand why! You gotta see her. My staff are pulling their hair out trying to settle her. We can hardly attend to anyone else! She's ringing the buzzer all the time, talking about some photographer – I really hope you can help us."

So here you are now in front of Mrs Constance, who looks like the queen as she sits regally in her bed telling you about, well, about – her words are clear but strange, "In the light of day I could see him standing there. There, just over there by the petunias." She points to a window with no view. "Snap! Snap! Snap! Went his camera and there was a scratching, it took me all over and then they got me! They tied me up by my hands and my feet and set fire to my bed. How can I forgive them for that? But, then again, the dogs that were standing beside them looked so lovely – so cute – they made me smile." What?! Did she know where she was and how she got here? Yes. Conversation moves wildly between the orientated and lucid to the extremely bizarre. But despite the fact that much of what she is saying sounds terrifying or – at best – haunting, Mrs Constance relays all of this to you in a monotone of calm. Is there an issue that she would like to explore? "Issues are the things of bitter bright lights that dance all around." Oh. Is she aware that she is constantly ringing the bell? "The nurses are the same as everyone. They need to know," and you politely thank Mrs Constance for answering your questions.

I am sure that you have guessed by now that Mrs Constance is not the type that one might usually see in an aged care facility. Perhaps she might have more in common with someone in a psychiatric ward.

But Mrs Constance came with no diagnosis of psychosis or history of psychiatrist intervention. How are staff to identify and manage someone at the far end of the mental health spectrum if they have had no training or experience in this area?

Addressing training and resource issues for aged care facilities are beyond the scope of this book, but it is enough to point out that staff tell me of the growing number of people they see whose needs are highly complex or ones that they are not familiar with. This experience is one that psychiatrists are both alert to and concerned about. They speak of "a rising tide" of older adults with psychiatric and general health concerns (Royal Australian and New Zealand College of Psychiatrists, calling for better coordination and resources for the over-65-year-old cohort; RANZCP 2010, p.2). In a later document the RANZCP specify the need to "improve the mental health of older people with distress or impairment related to functional and/or organic mental disorders" (RANZCP 2015, p.1) and be alert to concerns that mental illness is "common in elderly people, but often unrecognised by individuals, family and health care professionals, who may wrongly attribute symptoms of treatable mental illness to the irreversible effects of ageing or to physical or environmental changes" (RANZCP 2015, p.2).

An important part in psychotherapy with older adults is knowing the *limits* of your expertise and client suitability. This means that you need to be able to judge the difference between various presentations and assist staff with their options. It can be helpful, therefore, to see where mood or behaviour descriptors might be placed on the mental health and neurological spectrum so that the right care can be mobilized. Figure 4.1 details the three main stages of this spectrum and the associated examples of presentations.

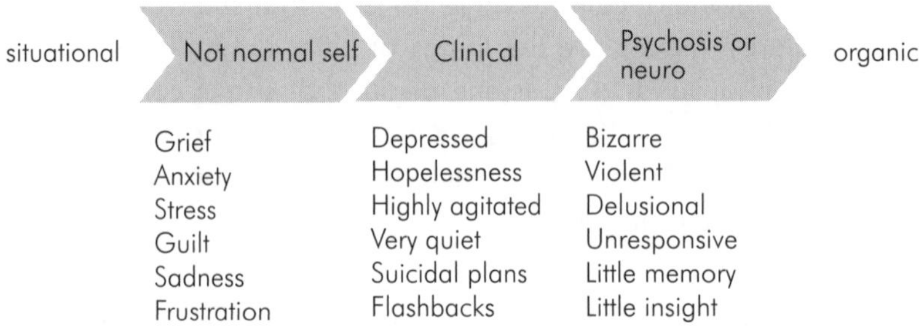

situational	Not normal self	Clinical	Psychosis or neuro	organic
	Grief	Depressed	Bizarre	
	Anxiety	Hopelessness	Violent	
	Stress	Highly agitated	Delusional	
	Guilt	Very quiet	Unresponsive	
	Sadness	Suicidal plans	Little memory	
	Frustration	Flashbacks	Little insight	

Figure 4.1: The mental health and neurological spectrum

At one end, the situational, staff might note that someone is not their usual self. They might also add that their husband has just died or their daughter has had to live interstate. When you talk more with the resident you discover grumblings of distress that may or may not be very evident to others. Distress may fluctuate and worsen but, overall, it is not severe enough to radically change their usual interests and is most likely related to a change of situation. In my opinion, prevention is better than cure so (if staff identify it soon enough or refer all new arrivals to you) this can be an ideal opportunity for you to normalize, listen and explore what changes have occurred.

In the middle of the spectrum are presentations that are more clinical in nature. Remember how Harold scored 27 out of 30 for the Geriatric Depression Scale? An outcome like that indicates a strong presence of depressive symptoms which would place him in the middle of this spectrum. While Harold might not have any history at all of depression or anxiety, others might have experienced a lifetime peppered with mental illness which means that there is a more stable component to their experience and they are more vulnerable to relapse. In Chapter 6 we will cover specific issues related to the lower and middle end of the spectrum like grief, pain, stress and trauma – all issues suitable for psychotherapeutic intervention.

Issues that are less suitable, or not relevant at all, are instances of extreme mental illness or neurological impairment where the person's capacity for change is unlikely or not possible. This usually relates to either a lifelong experience of illness or impairment, or a situation in which cognitive decline is marked. There might be an instance of intellectual impairment, severe stroke, neurological degeneration (alcohol abuse/Alzheimer's) or mental illness (schizophrenia/severe anxiety/bipolar affective disorder). In the case of older adults, physical ill-health or delirium is also likely and may be related to increased agitation. Table 4.1 offers a simple guide to differentiate between the main presentations that you are likely to see at the far end of the spectrum. Symptoms related to grief, associated with the lower to middle range, have also been included as a comparison.

Table 4.1: Delirium, delusion, dementia, depression and grief

Delirium[9]	Paranoia/ delusion	Dementia	Depression	Grief[10]
Sudden onset (e.g. urinary tract infection)	Fluctuating and often lifelong – but can present late in life	Gradual onset over several years	Fluctuating lifelong or over weeks after a life change	Specifically related to an experience of loss[11]
Fluctuating alertness and may appear very sleepy	Sometimes hyper-alert	Usually alert	Alert but often distant in engagement	Alert
Orientation often impaired	Orientation can fluctuate	Orientation often impaired and declines	Orientation normal	Orientation normal
Vivid and scary hallucinations likely	Rapid, bizarre or paranoid thoughts	Hallucinations possible	No hallucinations	No hallucinations
Distress likely to overshadow all else	Distress may block enjoyment	Can experience enjoyment	Sense of enjoyment impaired	Can experience enjoyment
Responsive to reason unlikely	Responsive to reason unlikely	Responsive to reason unlikely (e.g. late stages)	Responsive to reason blinkered	Responsive to reason
Mainly non-verbally agitated	Mainly verbally agitated	Agitation varies – can be aggressive	Low affect and not expressive	Emotionally expressive
May be fearful or angry	May be fearful or angry	May be fearful or angry	Angry at self and hopelessness felt	Specific guilt and temporary sadness
Temporary distress (days)	Persistent or cyclical distress	Persistent or cyclical distress	Chronic or temporary distress (months/years)	Temporary distress (months)

Information adapted or quoted from the following sources: Kessler 2015, p.22; Knight 2004, pp.124–130; and the NSW Department of Health 2006, pp.4–5 (reproduced by permission, NSW Department of Health © 2017). Please note that this reference is a simplified version of clinical sources and does not replace diagnostic assessment from a psychogeriatrician or geropsychologist.

The "5 Ps" of Cognitive Behavioural Therapy can be of added benefit in assessment: what are the presenting problems, the precipitating, perpetuating, predisposing and protective factors? Respectively, this translates to: what are your observations, issues that might have led up to the problem, what is maintaining it, the background dispositions, and responses (by self or others) that contain distress?

Determining suitability and whose problem it is

I invite you now to think back to Mrs Constance, and to consider the following: Is she suitable for psychotherapy? Whose problem is it mainly? How would you proceed? Before we examine the answers to these questions, here is the mental health and neurological spectrum again (Figure 4.2) but this time with a guide for deciding how to intervene.

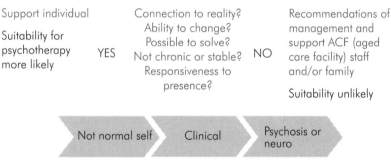

Figure 4.2: Initial determining of suitability

For Mrs Constance, I would not hesitate to suggest a referral to the Older Persons Mental Health Service. First, her needs are beyond the scope of a talking therapy where some level of reason is required. Second, her motivation to engage in a service is not likely to be high as, on the whole, she does not perceive herself to have a problem. Her delusions may be disturbing to her at times (certainly they are to others) and she may be highly engaging of staff but she does not appear overly concerned about her version of reality. She is certainly not bothered about how her behaviour is affecting others. As I am not a psychogeriatrician or a geropsychologist, I would recommend specialist assessment to address distress and get support for staff – who are the ones most affected by this problem.

What should be said, however, is that referrals to specialist services – whether they be for psychiatric concerns or dementia – do not always yield positive outcomes. Perhaps this is due to burgeoning need and few resources. Staff may complain to you that a response did not occur or that it was inadequate. The reality is that sometimes it falls back to facility staff to muddle through. While the needs of people with psychosis may be too great or beyond the scope of short-term psychological intervention, you can still be a support to staff.

Also, it is important not to dismiss those with a psychiatric diagnosis or mistake their ramblings for cognitive impairment (Knight 2004). I have worked with a number of people with a psychiatric diagnosis who have benefited from learning calming techniques. In instances where the older adult has received decades of psychiatric intervention, they may well be more expert than you in knowing what works and your role here is simply to facilitate this recall and encourage them to practise. Having strategies stuck on their wardrobe and sharing these with staff can further help manage ongoing cycles of distress.

In conclusion, the decision whether or not to continue seeing a client can be a difficult one. Factors such as responsiveness, current caseload, likelihood of progression, programme or funding criteria and whose problem it is all come into play. However, I would much rather have clinical discretion with these matters and scope to see clients informally (including staff and family) for a few sessions than a strict set of criteria. If there is distress, interest and some degree of responsiveness to supportive listening techniques then I believe psychotherapy should be seen as a viable option.

Many clients have had the edge taken off distress through some level of engagement – or by teaching staff how to support them. Unfortunately, however, this approach is not possible in government-rebated health systems where therapy is only available if the client is cognisant and interested enough to pursue a mental health care plan – and remember that they agreed to this. If this was a requirement for the current cohort of advanced seniors in residential settings that I see in one programme, then a minuscule number would receive the healing touch of psychotherapy. Even programmes where the intake funnel is currently wide run the risk of having to shrink programme criteria to step into line with generic funding guidelines that do not consider the unique considerations of effectively engaging advanced seniors (more about that in the final chapter). There are many shades of grey in determining suitability, but I believe that having flexibility in terms of who you support, and in what way, will ensure that more comprehensive and relevant intervention takes place.

Informal assessment

For those to whom you believe psychotherapy could be of benefit, there are a range of informal assessments that you can complete (on your own) to help you determine how to tailor intervention. Psychotherapy with older adults can be much like an elastic band: when ability, interest and circumstances are good it can be stretched out as wide as with any other population. When ability, interest and circumstances are challenged then it needs to contract in order to stay suitable for the unique needs of that individual or day.

Situations can change very dramatically for older adults, which is why continual assessment is so crucial. If delirium is present due to an infection then therapy needs to be suspended until the client recovers. If sight is becoming a problem, there is no point asking them to fill in worksheets. If hearing is an issue then it is inappropriate to conduct softly spoken meditation exercises. For intervention to be appropriate it needs to be relevant and flexible. Case conceptualization might need to be more of an ongoing process than with other population groups. The following is a list of questions I have devised that you can rate out of 10 or answer as low, medium, high or unsure. The full sheet can be found in Appendix 1.

1. How much is the problem their problem?

2. How much is the problem someone else's, e.g. facility, another resident, family?

3. What is their ability to engage like? Consider sight, memory, insight, concentration or fatigue, comprehension, hearing, speech, hand dexterity, overall mobility, level of pain or discomfort, external distractions (neighbours/TV) and irritations, level of privacy and degree to which staff respect "therapy in progress" signs.

4. How motivated are they to change or take responsibility for their concerns?

5. How able are they to change? Do they have an intellectual impairment or dementia?

6. How familiar are they with the concept of counselling?

7. How complex or severe is the presenting problem?

8. What are their external supports like and how able are they to access them?

9. How concerned are they about how they are perceived by others in accessing your support? Are they worried about privacy or stigma issues?

10. How comfortable are they in discussing their personals with you? Do you need to provide extra comfort here in terms of understanding generational difference?

Formal assessment

Depending on your discipline and theoretical orientation, how much you rely on formal assessment will vary. You also might be required by the organization you work for to carry out a routine set of assessment scales that are usually linked to funding. The issue of what type of formal assessment to deliver, when, how or if at all is a thorny issue sure to create division. I am neither anti formal assessment nor embracing of it to the extent that it is often used. The following is a brief description of formal assessments that I have used and why I have found them helpful. Then I will discuss assessments that I believe are unsuitable for a large number of seniors, followed by concerns about the general reliance on formal assessments.

The Mini Mental State Examination

This type of assessment is very good as a dementia screening tool (Knight 2004) and I have found it particularly helpful for presentations that are less common than Alzheimer's disease. When dementia is undiagnosed this tool can be helpful in suggesting to medical staff and family that behaviour or issues could be neurologically based and warrant more thorough investigation. If it is frontotemporal dementia then impaired logic and reasoning may lead to misunderstandings and high emotion. Family might feel offended and not realize that their otherwise lucid parent has cognitive deficits. If it is vascular dementia then damage can be very diffuse, depending on the areas affected, and if damage is still occurring (i.e. a bleed) then cognitive impairment will accumulate. It is worth pointing out here that while it might be commonplace for residents to be screened when admitted to a facility, there is usually no yearly review of such status; therefore, decline can go undetected. Mostly it would be hard to justify the expense and human resource to routinely assess a resident's cognitive status because usually staff can see the common signs of decline and adjust – except when the presentation is not so common.

This reminds me of one chap for whom it was known that he had experienced multiple transient ischaemic attacks or mini strokes. Staff had referred him because they and his wife were finding him to be "very difficult" with activities of daily living such as dressing and eating. Could I help? He was a retired bus driver and my initial visit was in his room with his wife present. He appeared able to comprehend well enough – he could answer closed questions at least – and he looked alert and engaged. Would he mind if I sat here and asked him a few questions? "No, that's fine," he said. Is it okay if his wife stays in the room while I speak to him? "Oh, yes. I'd like her to be here," he offered while giving her an appreciative glance.

But with his wife there I did not get to hear much from him. She did most of the talking and he deferred to her regularly. "Always been like that!" she laughed, aware of this long-standing ritual. "Yes," my client agreed, "it has." Then his wife added, "He's never been much of a talker," which was followed by him replying, "No, that's true, I haven't." Nothing appeared obviously awry but I felt the need to see him on his own, would they mind? That had them both looking worried but they consented.

This next session shed a very different light. First, I noted that after only one week there was no recognition of who I was. Then there was the difficulty answering open-ended questions which were mostly followed with "Oh, I don't know" type answers. He was not sure how long he had been at the facility, did not furnish with much detail about life before moving in, was not able to name any of those who smiled back at him in the photos on the wall (much to his consternation), and often looked at me blankly as if he had lost the thread of where our conversation was going. But what had me most amazed was how difficult it was for him to answer a very simple five-scale set of questions – the Emotion Thermometers Tool – which is discussed in the next section. It took a good part of the session for me to try different tack after different tack but he was only able to answer two out of the five questions. And it did not seem as though he did not want to give an answer; it was more that he could not.

There was nothing very startling about his score on the Psychogeriatric Assessment Scales, which "…is designed to gather information on the major psychogeriatric disorders: dementia and depression" (Jorm and Mackinnon 1995, p.5), and was administered two years ago upon admission. So, no diagnosis of dementia. His wife had complained that one of the things she finds most frustrating is that he just refuses to eat. "I'll ask him to put another mouthful of food in and then he'll just stop again! So, I have to ask again! It's driving me crazy. I don't know why he's being so difficult," she confided. If you are assuming that someone has remembered what you have just said then this would indeed seem like they are refusing in some way; being difficult. But what if they had not remembered? Time for some exploration.

His score on the Mini Mental State Examination was 20 out of 30 which, overall, is said to increase the odds that dementia is present and suggests mild cognitive impairment. But, while a score like this suggests some abnormality for someone who has completed an eighth grade education, in an overall sense it did not suggest a huge problem. What appeared more of a problem to me was this chap's complete inability to get most of the orientation questions right and not being able to score at all on the delayed recall item. Was he still experiencing multiple transient ischaemic attacks (undetected) which was effectively wiping out his short-term memory? Only a more thorough cognitive assessment by someone like a psychogeriatrician would be able to give an answer on this one. But his medical practitioner did not agree with me. "I don't see any point in doing that," he said, "he does not seem too agitated to me." No, the resident was not agitated – he probably just forgets – but everyone else around him was! Times like these can be frustrating but there was no going forward if the GP was putting his foot down. What ended up being helpful, however, was to present a theory of short-term memory loss to his wife and staff and suggest radical changes in expectations. This seemed to do the trick and led me to see his wife on her own – not for frustration now but for grief.

The Emotion Thermometers Tool[12]

This is my all-time favourite. It was created by Dr Alex J. Mitchell in 2007, initially for use in oncology, and is an adaptation of the American Distress Thermometer (University of Leicester 2017). It is easy to use even when there are significant ability issues present. When completing this simple five-question visual analogue scale takes almost an entire session, like in the example above, then that is also useful information! The scale is from 0 to 10 and ranges from "extreme" to "not at all". The questions, for most clients, are easily understood and having thermometers for each variable gives this clinically validated tool a more user-friendly feel. Also the speech impaired can point out their answers and it is a form that is not very intimidating so can be done even when rapport is being developed, sometimes even before formal sessions have commenced. The first measure alone – distress – can get to the heart of how much your client believes that they have a problem. Sometimes I use the word "sadness" instead of depression and "frustration" instead of anger so clients, especially advanced seniors who are women, can relate better to what I am asking them. This can also be a good tool to review therapy and/or for evaluating therapy effectiveness. However, for reasons that I will discuss in Chapter 9, relying on such quantitative measures has limitations when it comes to an advanced senior clientele.

The Geriatric Depression Scale

By now you are probably a little familiar with this scale. You might remember that in the preface Mary scored high on this scale but then went on to respond very well to psychotherapy. Think, too, of Harold and the responses he gave when we were exploring psychological distress in Chapter 3. Despite the fact that I am not a fan of the term "geriatric" and never refer to its full name with clients, this tool has been designed specifically for use with an older population by Yesavage et al. (1983) and can accurately assess for the presence of depressive symptoms which may then require a medication review request. The "yes" or "no" answers allow for ease of answering when cognitive co-morbidities are present. However, despite its simple format, sometimes extra explanations are required, breaks between questions needed, or gentle re-direction provided to bring your client back to the question list. There is also a shorter version of this scale

(Yesavage 1988). The recently developed Geriatric Anxiety Inventory by Pachana *et al.* (2007) is an easy to use 20-item questionnaire that also is available in a five-item version (Byrne and Pachana 2011).

The Intake Form

This form can be found in Appendix 2. I designed this questionnaire because I could not find anything else that adequately guided conversation in a semi-focused manner. It is not an empirically designed instrument – it has not been clinically tested or validated – and I doubt if it should ever be used for this purpose. The answers are less about the clinician arriving at some sort of judgement, and more a means for client insight and co-consultation of the problem. I use it mainly when distress is evident to me but there is reluctance to talk or perhaps a lack of awareness about why they are feeling the way they do or what issues are present that could benefit from psychotherapy.

Sometimes I complete the page of questions in one session but mostly I let questions be a springboard to them telling me their story and having an experiential understanding of how counselling can facilitate relief. For example, just the question "Are you missing your pets?" can uncover a whole world of grief and mixed memories. One note of caution: never literally read the questions out as is but weave them into a question that is relevant to your particular client. For example, instead of "Are you grieving the loss or decline of your spouse?" ask "I remember you telling me a bit about Mavis. When you've been married for that long it can be perfectly natural to miss things about that person that aren't there as much now. Dementia has changed the way Mavis is a lot hasn't it? I wonder if you find yourself missing the Mavis you once knew at times?" So, you see, these questions are more just a guide for you to incorporate your own clinical judgement in how you phrase them to your clients.

As well as working with seniors, I work with a range of other clients or issues in both a salaried position and in private practice: adults of various ages, carers, people with life-limiting illness, trauma, new mothers and people with a disability. What often amazes me is how easily *all* of these clients are able to answer various questionnaires as opposed to advanced seniors. Not only are there less complicating issues (hearing loss, etc.) but also there appears to be an acceptance of this process and a willingness to "behave" in a way that allows you to get to the end as quickly as possible. At worst, a client of a younger group may appear bored with the process but is very rarely (if at all) highly suspicious or incapable of giving a straight answer. It is as if they have been socialized into accepting that one must answer a battery of personal questions if one is to access emotional support. Whether this is a good thing or a bad thing will depend on your personal orientation.

What I have discovered is that advanced seniors can be delightfully non-conformist – some might say resistant – to giving expedient answers to questions on a form. It is as if they are defining on their own terms what is and what is not important. Yes, this can be frustrating, but it highlights to me a couple of issues that I will explore with you now: senior-friendly *measures* in formal assessment and senior-friendly *approaches*.

Senior-friendly *measures* in formal assessment

Have you ever used the Kessler Psychological Distress Scale (K10)? In clinical circles it is often viewed as a simple (too simple some might say) measure of ten questions to discover the presence and extent of depression and anxiety symptoms. Questions like "About how often did you feel depressed?" and options such as "a little of the time" or "most of the time" are usually navigated with ease. For advanced seniors, however, having a range of five response options can throw them into confusion. Or they may simply not understand some of the terminology used or become defensive in their answers.

Other more complicated (and more comprehensive) measures like the Depression Anxiety and Stress Scale (DASS) may be unwittingly used by either doctors or clinicians and result in greater distress. Many such measures can be inappropriate for older adults (Pachana *et al.* 2010) so it is vitally important, in my opinion, that the measures you use relate well to this population group. Even tools that have been designed for seniors may not be useful for *advanced* seniors. Once such example is the California Older Person's Pleasant Events Schedule designed by Rider, Gallagher-Thompson and Thompson (2004). The idea behind this tool is admirable. Clearly influenced by the positive psychology movement, the question process appears to be designed to illuminate enjoyable activities and stimulate discussion about how to re-incorporate these activities if they have become neglected.

This goal is congruent with depression management too – encourage simple mastery skills to develop a sense of achievement, stimulate mood through behavioural activation, increase a sense of personal autonomy, and feel better about life through engaging in pleasant events.

The only thing is that there are 66 questions with six different response options for each question. For seniors who like to tell a story at many points along the way, or have communication issues, this questionnaire can take a number of sessions! Also, for advanced seniors, it can stimulate grief more than anything because even the simple act of looking at clouds might well be a pastime they once enjoyed but can no longer do if they are sight impaired. I imagine that it is probably more appropriate in general for the medium-old who need a gentle reminder about all the things that they still can do and who are able to complete this inventory on their own.

Senior-friendly approaches in formal assessment

I believe that an important question before administering any form of assessment is: Why? This is as relevant for seniors as it is for any population. What is it that you are wanting to discover? Is it what your client is interested in? Could the outcome expand their options or negatively impact self-esteem? What could be the benefit in learning more? What could be the disadvantages? What other agendas are there in gaining this understanding: adhering to risk management guidelines, aiming for positive pre/post scores, funding requirements, habit, keeping professional integrity, interests in following "best practice" as determined by research with other populations?

Is it possible that sometimes an interest in conducting formal assessment might be one small step away from what the client really wants – needs – and one closer to an anxiety about not being good enough? Not thorough enough? Not scientific enough? I realize that these questions might be contentious but my concern here is an apparent over-active interest in clinical circles with psychological measures and how this could damage rapport in the initial phases of seeing a senior – not to mention their already flailing identity as an able person. From my consultations with older adults it is apparent that they already feel like a group of medicalized parts. Do we really need to be another professional who seems more interested in their pathology than them as a person? It is not that I am opposed to a level of investigation about pathology. Discerning the difference between a treatable mental or medical condition and a presentation that is more related to cognitive impairment is critical to valuing the rights that an older adult has to having quality of life. Investigations that seek to gain an accurate understanding of the causes behind distress can be extremely beneficial to all concerned – client, family and staff.

But equally critical is exercising caution in if, when and what formal psychological assessments be used. Psychologists themselves have expressed concern that their general training in clinical service provision "portrays them as the expert" (APS 2000, p.28) and that this approach can undermine effectiveness with an older adult population. Assuming the position of "expert" can, I believe, limit empowering practices that give space for client self-definition – viewing the person's situation in ways that are useful to the client and not in ways that science deems "correct" or that relate more to an agenda the therapist has. In social work there are strong values and ethics like beneficence and non-malfeasance that guide research and practice (Antle and Regehr 2003). Care needs to be taken that psychotherapeutic interactions with seniors, especially in relation to assessments, do not unwittingly create a disempowering context.

While I am appreciative of the contributions of science and geropsychology, as a mental health social worker I am also influenced by my profession's code of ethics (Australian Association of Social Workers 2010). I am also influenced by the philosophy of Narrative Therapy which rejects an expert stance (Bubenzer, West and Boughner 1995) and actively deconstructs knowledge practices by viewing clients as the "primary authors of these knowledges and practices" (White 1992, p.144). It might be helpful to clarify here that this does not mean that someone cannot be considered an expert in their field, but that in their interactions with clients they are not assuming to be the expert of that person's life based on their own suspicions or on what the science might suggest. My interest is in a psychotherapeutic practice that is neither too medical and focused on pathology or the science, nor ignorant of a clinical outlook and the evidence base available. I also believe that this "middle way" approach, when applied to seniors, offers an engagement strategy that is person centred vs disease focused and keeps a watchful eye for subtle forms of maleficence mentioned earlier in Chapter 2. By all means use formal assessments, but please, do so with much thought and caution. And, as the following chapter will discuss, developing connection may trump anything else that happens to be in your clinician's toolbox.

PERSONAL REFLECTION

1. What did you find most interesting about this chapter?

_____

_____

2. What knowledge did you already have that was reinforced for you?

_____

_____

3. How many of the formal assessment measures were you already familiar with? Which ones were they?

_____

_____

4. How do you feel about formal assessments?

_____

_____

5. What things would you like to be most mindful of when you consider the issue of assessment for older adults?

_____

_____

CHAPTER 5

INVITATIONS FOR ENGAGEMENT

When I tap on a resident's door to meet them for the first time I always expect the unexpected. What I find and what transpires as I respond to a "Yes...?" on the other side is like the mixing of musical chords – the possibilities are endless. Remember that for the majority of my facility referrals the clients are unsuspecting. There can be good reason for this – facility staff are not always the best ones to broach the concept of counselling. The way that your service is explained and how you engage in your initial contact can "make or break" the likelihood of a resident continuing and benefiting from psychotherapy.

So, rather deliberately, my first visit is usually a surprise. This can be the case even when my private service is accessed and residents have agreed to a mental health care plan. How much they understood about what was on offer when talking with their doctor and how personally invested in it they are is often another story. They may not be interested in when the appointment was scheduled, not had staff remind them, or forgotten even when they were told. While first appointments with seniors in the community (home visiting or centre based) can still be occasions where clients do not seem to know what is going on, this is all the more the case when responding to a facility referral.

I treasure these moments – these first glimpses of who has been referred to you – for they can hold within them an explosion of learning and engagement opportunity. I find it enthralling, if not a little exhausting at times. There can be a lot to take in, a lot to navigate. They may be friendly, apathetic, hostile, dismissive, wary, deflecting, and a whole range of other variables mentioned earlier that can make up this experience, and also determine whether or not psychotherapy is suitable in this instance. This encounter can unlock a world of understanding and allow you to, as clinical psychologist Dr Paul Bogenberger (2014) suggests, "talk to your client before they are a client". Seeing them as a person first, not a referral or a client, is vitally important. This goes beyond client-centred work, beyond the frame of "client" and considers the human before you. Just as Chapter 2 discusses barriers to engagement, this chapter explores how engagement can be created.

The missing jigsaw piece

The idea that sessions, especially initial ones, sensitively engage older adults is not novel. For example, Knight (2004) discusses the importance of adapting the environment to maximize comfort, communicating in a way that overcomes developmental changes or disability, actively orientating seniors to the psychotherapeutic process, demonstrating an interest in their unique perception, being familiar with cohort influences and seeking to learn about their broader context. As with any initial therapeutic encounter, physical accessibility, effective communication, clarifying the service, developing understanding, rapport and trust are all pillars for successful engagement.

However, when clients have not self-referred or when they are largely uninvested in the referral then the process of engagement is even more delicate and it is not a process that appears to be dealt with sufficiently in the literature. How do you successfully engage an advanced senior in care who has not self-referred but who, for all intents and purposes, is a good candidate for psychotherapy? How do you reduce the risk of refusal through mismanagement? The answer to this, I believe, is the missing jigsaw piece to completing the picture of psychotherapeutic work with older adults.

Mrs Need: [tone is wary] Yes? Hello…

Therapist: [opening the door wider] Ah, hello, Mrs Need?

Mrs Need: Yes dear.

Therapist: Hi, my name is Lucy and – do you mind if I sit down? [Mrs Need nods in approval but looks a little suspicious] Thank you. I'm a therapist from the Sunnyday Counselling Service.

Mrs Need: [looks at therapist blankly]

Therapist: The nurses thought you might be interested in our service. They said that you had been having a lot of trouble sleeping lately and were a bit teary –

Mrs Need: Oh, it's nothing dear. Just old age I guess –

Therapist: Just because people are your age doesn't mean they should put up with not sleeping well or having low mood. Sometimes people of your age have what's called anxiety or depression, but it's treatable and that's where I come in.

Mrs Need: [smiles but still looks wary] Well, that's very kind of you dear but I'm not sure that I can help you.

Therapist: Well, it's not about you helping me, it's about me helping you. [hands her a brochure] See, this explains more about our service. Psychological intervention can be very helpful for people at any age who are experiencing problems – like not sleeping properly, feeling uptight or feeling sad all the time. Why don't I pop by in a fortnight's time to see if you're interested?

Mrs Need: Oh, I don't know if I have any real problems.

Therapist: [tone is encouraging] You don't have to be a part of the service but it could help.

Mrs Need: [sounds unsure] Well, okay.

Do you think that Mrs Need is going to take up Lucy's offer? How about another example?

Mrs Need: [tone is wary] Yes? Hello…

Therapist: [opening the door wider] Ah, hello, Mrs Need?

Mrs Need: Yes dear.

Therapist: Goodness! [looking at quilt on the bed]. What a gorgeous quilt [an authentic compliment]. Did you make it?

Mrs Need: Yes dear [smiles].

Therapist: It's so intricate. Have you always had an interest in quilting?

Mrs Need: I used to be a seamstress.

Therapist: Oh, I see, well you probably have a good eye for quality workmanship then?

Mrs Need: [looks down at gnarly hands] Yes. Not that that's much use to me now.

Therapist: [indicating to the spare chair] Do you mind? [Mrs Need nods but looks wary] Sorry, my name's Lucy and I spend a lot of time listening to people around your age. What seems to come out more than anything are how many changes that can happen, things that maybe even have you not feeling like yourself anymore. Would you say that that's been the case for you a bit?

Mrs Need: Well, yes, a bit, but I'm fine, really.

Therapist: [mock horror] I haven't even told you where I'm from! [hands her a brochure] I do something called counselling. Most people I see don't know much about it but that's okay. It's often a case of just "dipping your toe" in and seeing if it's something that you think could be helpful. It can be especially helpful when a lot of changes have gone on – moving into a facility, moving away from your home, changes to your body – things like that. It's not like everything is all bad. Many people I speak to are quite appreciative of a lot of things – it's just that counselling can give you a chance to talk about things that you might not normally be able to. After all, staff are usually pretty busy, aren't they?

Mrs Need: Yes.

Therapist: [looking back at the quilt] Tell me more about your seamstress days. Do you know, I'm all fingers and thumbs when it comes to sewing. [Mrs Need smiles and speaks of the things she used to make and how colleagues became lifelong friends]

Mrs Need: But Bonnie died a few years ago.

Therapist: You miss her?

Mrs Need: [with tears in her eyes] Oh yes, terribly. [brushing off the low mood] Oh! She was such a bright spark! [She glances at a ledge of photos]

Therapist: Is that her over there? [Mrs Need nods and therapist takes a closer look] Sounds like you were two peas in a pod! [Mrs Need smiles wistfully] What is it that Bonnie liked about being around you, do you think?

Mrs Need: [tone bashful] Oh, I don't know. I made her laugh I guess. And I'd been sewing longer that she'd been so she came to me for help and things.

Therapist: There's that eye for detail and quality again! [Mrs Need smiles appreciatively] So, look, there's no pressure [looking to the brochure in Mrs Need's hand] but staff often tell me when they think someone doesn't seem like themselves and my job is to meet with them and let them make up their own mind as to whether getting some counselling could help. Like I said, often it's just a case of dipping your toe in first so you can see for yourself. Like, even just now. What's it been like telling me about Bonnie and your sewing days?

Mrs Need: Oh, well, sad I guess, but also good [smiles warmly].

Therapist: There you go. Maybe this counselling thing could be worth a shot, eh?

Mrs Need: I guess [returns Lucy's smile and says sincerely]. Thank you.

Which Lucy of these two examples do you think Mrs Need has warmed to the most? And which of these two "Lucys" is Mrs Need likely to agree continuing with? You guessed it. Chances are that the counsellor in the second example is the one that Mrs Need will be most comfortable with and eventually open up to a discussion about the symptoms that she has been experiencing lately. Did you notice, too, how in the second example Mrs Need seemed to say "yes" more often? Many moons ago I was a sales assistant and we were taught that eliciting a "yes" is more likely to secure a sale. Generally I baulk at this type of coercion, especially if it relates to making money (my sales career had a short life), but I do not mind drawing on a little psychology of influence if it is to help people feel more comfortable accessing a service that could benefit them.

Did you also notice how Lucy, second time around, did not mention anything about symptoms but instead spoke about change and how conversation seemed to naturally turn to Mrs Need sharing some of her distress? The "second" Lucy also did lots of affirming of Mrs Need as a person and zeroed in on her abilities. Later on in therapy Mrs Need might be more receptive to grief therapy in relation to multiple loss. Conversations could also capitalize on how Mrs Need appeared to accept that she did have a good eye for detail and quality. Maybe this aspect about her identity could become enlarged in therapy and links could be made to values that are ever strong in her despite diminished capacity. Perhaps she could be encouraged to participate in judging at the annual craft fair? She might not be able to produce the same work as before but she might still be able to be admired for her clever eye. Yes, fears would need to be addressed, confidence built and other needs met, but when people are looked at as people first and foremost then the emphasis on engagement is not on deficit and symptoms but on resources and abilities. Dignity and human connection become more paramount than correction and an explicit helper role.

Undercover agents

Call this type of engagement crafty if you like, but what is the alternative? Alienation because the therapist is just coming in with their own idea of what helping looks like? I prefer not to see such intervention as crafty but consultative. You give yourself time to see things from Mrs Need's point of view. You consult her on what she holds as important in her life – past and present. You discover how things have changed for her before rushing in with descriptors that she has not used to define her experience. You explore with her what her experience is of anything that she wishes to talk about. You listen to her as a human being before you even see her as a client.

Through careful attention paid to interests and exceptions of moments where distress was less, little by little, you invite Mrs Need into a therapeutic relationship that honours who she is more than what she is not. Your reward after such sensitive navigation is a firm foundation of trust onto which you can build all manner of interventions to address the problems that are now freely being identified. To help you do this, here are five guiding principles that you can refer to when you are first meeting with an advanced senior:

1. *Dignity* How can you build them up? (Not in a patronizing or unauthentic way.)

2. *Choice* How can you help them feel like they are in control of the process?

3. *Value* What is it about their conversation that speaks of important values?

4. *Trust* What opportunities are there to reaffirm their trust in you?

5. *Permission to talk* How can you comfortably invite them into conversation?

Yes, a lot can ride on that first meet. Sometimes it will not work out. Sometimes, despite your best efforts, they will decline. All this is perfectly okay. Maybe they do not need the service. What is most important is that you try to free yourself from the cobwebs of agenda and just relax into your interest of this person as a human being.

The Life Story Interview[13]

If you want to know me, you must know my story, for my story defines who I am. (Dan McAdams 1993, quoted in Moore, Metcalf and Schow 2000)

In the introduction of this book I shared how I began my psychotherapeutic work with older adults in care. At the time, my colleague and I were still unaware of Reminiscence Therapy, Dignity Therapy or Life Review work. In hindsight knowledge of these theories would have made navigating therapeutic engagement a little more easy with a population who appeared to be of a very different ilk to others we had worked with. But not being aware of practices commonplace in this field was a blessing in disguise I believe. It meant that we pursued with great vigour how best to intervene. We were hungry for a system of thought and practice that allowed us to be therapeutically relevant and sensitive. Nothing in our immediate network satiated this hunger so, with an interest in consulting from a person-centred framework, it seemed perfectly natural to focus our attention on the older adult themselves: observe, learn and discover all that we could about their multi-storied lives and what was most important to them.

While the new programme we were operating under was developed specifically to address the emotional and psychological needs of residents in care, there were very few parameters. On the one hand this was disconcerting, but on the other it gave us freedom to experiment.

We did not need to distinguish between informal or formal sessions, there were no pre/post measures to fill out; there were no forms at all. All that was required was that the general practitioner consented to us intervening with their patient – in time we were able to rearrange this to an emphasis toward client consent. Our foray into this new world also took us deep into a land of reflective practice and had us arriving at the following conclusions.

Residents were often wary about counselling and seemed to not feel worthy

Most were wary about the counselling process. They appeared to know little of what "counselling" or "wellbeing" meant and seemed uncomfortable with the idea of being helped. It also appeared that they did not feel worthy of receiving help or felt shame about receiving it. These reactions led us to wondering how their history might have fostered a steely resilience to cope with difficult times and how we could encourage them to engage with us without "losing face" or be seen as weak. Perhaps cohort influences were at play here, as in the collective disposition of "the lucky generation".

We also wondered about the part that our society might be playing in revering its youth more than its aged and the potential to feel "forgotten" after becoming a facility resident. Often detached from the community and no longer seen as productive, our Western culture can prize productivity and youth over age and wisdom. These were all subtle messages that we thought could have a senior believe that they were not worthy of being listened to. It was not uncommon that seniors who had been referred did not know how to initiate a conversation about a "problem", but they could become engaged in a process of story telling, and from that often acknowledged present-day concerns.

Residents often expressed a desire to be helpful

Another theme that emerged was that they often replied to suggestions of telling their story with, "If that is helpful for you dear…" So I started to wonder what it would be like if counselling could take place in the context of them telling their story and for them to have the perception of being helpful. My colleague liked this idea and we explored how an interviewing process denotes some need for the interviewee to help the "reporter" gather important elements of a story. The story was the resident's life: their past, present and future and all that it meant to them. When we tried this out residents appeared more comfortable being able to help in this way – that it was about them helping us, not us helping them – and seemed to give them a greater sense of value and purpose. From these conversations rapport was easily built and most times questions that were asked as a conversation stimulant ended up becoming a springboard into more formal and explicit therapy encounters.

Residents appeared to feel invisible

Residents often reported (and still do to me) that they feel like just a number when in a facility setting. The interview process became for us an informal and non-threatening way to uncover "lost selves" – selves that had become invisible during the ageing process and living in a facility context. It seemed to be a way of "pulling them out of the rubble" and seeing them as the person they really are. It was also a way for women, especially, to celebrate parts of themselves that were not ordinarily acknowledged in terms of success or achievement regarding their unpaid work endeavours.

From these conclusions we developed an interview pro forma which has an interest not only to engage the resident in conversation but also to create opportunities for seniors to re-author their histories in ways that are more invigorating and useful for them. There are nine main questions in the Life Story Interview and multiple sub-questions which can be varied according to the individual and circumstance. Topics covered include questions about childhood, youth, relationships, significant events (enjoyable and difficult), loss, self-image, love and conflicts, meaning making, interests in reconnection and their legacy for future generations. There is no strict order, it is often best to move from one topic to the other as the story flows, but having some format can make it more comfortable for client and therapist (interviewee and interviewer) to proceed when the senior is wary of counselling or not forthcoming with their story.

1. Important people
Who have been, or still are, the special people in your life? Why are they important to you?

2. Growing up: childhood and early adult years

Where were you born? What memories stand out the most for you when you remember your childhood and early adult years? Do certain toys, pets, people or events come to mind? Are there aspects of the Depression and World War II that impacted you and have stayed in your consciousness?

3. Family: children

Are there any aspects about your own children and/or children who were important to you – e.g. nieces or nephews – that you would like to share? This could be both events that have happened in the past or interesting facts about the present such as where they live and what they do. Are there any memories that make you smile?

4. Family: parents and elders

Who were you most close to growing up? Did you have a favourite parent, aunt/uncle or grandparent? What did you admire the most about them? Can you share some memories about what this special person did to include you in their life? What did this mean to you? What might it have meant for this person to know you? Were there aspects of your life that this person seemed to appreciate the most – qualities they seemed most taken by or enjoyed? How would you describe the connection that you shared and how it featured in your life, what it meant to you?

Were there any relationships with parents or elders that were difficult? What aspects about these relationships bothered you the most? What do you wish was different? Do strong feelings about this/these relationship(s) still overshadow your life in some respects? Is this something that you are comfortable with? If there was one thing that you would like to work through in terms of these difficult memories or experiences then what would it be or whom would it be about? What capabilities might the special person you mentioned earlier have appreciated about your ability to try and manage the challenges associated with this difficult family member – or with any life difficulty that you have experienced?

5. Family: brothers, sisters and others

What memories do you have about your brothers, sisters, cousins or any other relative? How do you feel about these relationships now?

6. Interests, hobbies and recreational activities

Did you play sport at any stage in your life? Were you good at what you did? Did you go to dances when you were younger? What interests or activities have been most important to you over the years? These might be things that you did when you were in your teens, it might be something that you have kept going for a while, it might be something that you commenced in retirement, or it might even be something that you are enjoying now. Do you enjoy listening to music? What songs did you or do you like listening to? Is there a certain place or situation where you most enjoyed listening to this music like in the car? Did you sing songs around the piano? What were your favourite songs? Have you got a special song that reminds you of someone or something? Have you ever tried singing it? Is there a song or type of music that makes you feel good?

7. Community contributions and occupational work

Looking back over your life, what activities (paid or unpaid), occupied a lot of your time and contributed to either your family or society? This might be raising children, volunteer work or professional work. What was important about this work? What did you enjoy the most about doing it and what achievements are you most proud of? If other people were to do this type of work or activity, what key characteristics or values do you think that they would need to have?

8. Themes of your life: values and characteristics

Looking back over all of your life, are there certain themes that come through? What metaphors would you use to describe your life? If your story were a novel, for instance, then what would the "chapters" be about? Would there be an overall theme of your life or maybe a mixture of themes like "a comedy", "a tragedy", "a mystery", "a romance"? Are there any aspects of these chapters that you would like to reflect more on? If you had your time again would you want to change or expand anything? What are the most important roles that you've played in your life? What are you most proud of? What might others say about someone who took that approach? How might they describe them? What traits best describe the person you are, i.e. hard working, caring, strong, trusting, independent, optimistic, loving, brave, mischievous, cooperative, humorous, creative, friendly, courageous, shy? When you think back to difficult times, what characteristics did you draw on the most? Who in your life most witnessed these characteristics?

9. Memories: life now and legacies for the future

Is there a special image or place that you enjoy thinking about? What memories about your life do you value the most? Have you got an item or belonging that you particularly cherish? Why is it significant? What are you most grateful for in life? What would you say are your core beliefs or values that you like to live by? What do you value the most about your life now despite the changes and limitations that have been placed on you? What do you like the most about being the age you are now? What do you like the least? How would you like people, especially your family, to remember you? If there was one bit of advice you could give to the younger generation today, what would it be?

After reading this, you might rightly ask yourself, "Well, how different is that to Reminiscence Therapy, Dignity Therapy or Life Review work? Is this just 'reinventing the wheel'?" If so, then it is something that I have also wondered about since becoming more familiar with models intended to access life histories and facilitate a discussion on legacy. There certainly are similarities. But I believe that there are also subtle but important differences. If you imagine the evaluative reminiscence style that Dr Robert Butler developed at one end of a spectrum – older adults sharing stories with others in a group (Gerfo 1980) – and the 68 questions that comprise Barbara Haight's (1982) *Life Review and Experiencing Form* at the other, then the Life Story Interview would sit in the middle.

Dignity Therapy is at this middle point too of combining a pro forma with free-flowing exploration. Questions such as "Tell me a little about your life history, particularly the parts that you either remember most, or think are the most important. When did you feel most alive?" and "What are your most important accomplishments, and what do you feel most proud of?" (Dignity in Care 2016) appear identical. However, the express purpose of Dignity Therapy is for palliative contexts and the process typically involves just one session.

The Life Story Interview can be organized or free-flowing, stay at the interview level or be a conversational stimulant into deeper psychotherapeutic work. Perhaps the *practice* might be more similar to other life history work but the *objectives* are often different.

Table 5.1 spells this out in more detail and uses the *Life Review and Experiencing Form* as the main example for comparison.

Table 5.1: Life Story Interview in contrast with the Life Review and Experiencing Form

Similarities	Differences
Uses open-ended questions for life reflection	Intentionally uncovers "lost selves"
Facilitates emotional expression	Deeper work in identity reconnection
Builds a bridge from past to present	Not intended to be explored sequentially
Seeks to integrate past and create meaning	Not structured over a series of sessions
Consults the client on their interpretation	Only structured if the client is not leading
Brings new understandings and perspectives	Specifically draws on Narrative Therapy
Is an intentional exploration of story	Encourages the use of metaphor in reflection
For self-use or facilitated by a paraprofessional	For use only by trained counsellors
Could stimulate the recall of positive memories	Can be used just as a rapport stimulant
Could alleviate boredom and distress/regret	A platform to interweave other modalities
Could increase gratitude and decrease despair	Could result in a therapy document for client
Could result in a legacy document for family	Encourages moving back and forth in topic
A way to honour/acknowledge loss or difficulty	Exploration of client knowledges to deal with present context of distress
Offers a structured interviewing process	

With strong flavours of Narrative Therapy, and echoes of Rogerian philosophy, the overarching interest in the Life Story Interview is that the senior feels invited to share their multi-storied life in a way that opens up possibilities for them rich with meaning and acknowledgement and which facilitates personal agency. Like the narrative metaphor in Narrative Therapy, the Life Story Interview engages with life histories in a way that encourages the construction of positive change and identity. Specifically it relates to this intent of a narrative practice:

> Re-authoring conversations re-invigorate people's efforts to under-stand what it is that is happening in their lives, what it is that has happened, how it has happened, and what it all means. In this way, these conversations encourage a dramatic re-engagement with life and with history, and provide options for people to more fully inhabit their lives and their relationships... It is in this dramatic re-engagement that the gaps in the story line are filled. (White 2005, p.10)

Such conversations also reinforce the senior as the expert in their own life – having their own unique knowledges – which I think is a wonderful antidote to imbalances that can occur in clinical settings where knowledge and power are synonymous forces that centre around the role of the practitioner.

Given the multiple ways that the Life Story Interview can be implemented, and the many different tracks of conversation that might result from this engagement, it should not be seen as simply a recollection or retelling tool that anyone (e.g. a trained volunteer) can do. It is a model which is full of psychotherapeutic intent. Not only can it be therapeutic in and of itself, but it can allow for a stepped approach to intervention where therapeutic intensity can escalate according to needs the therapist becomes aware of through their observational or listening skills. For example, suppose you were listening to a senior recount their childhood and they pause and turn away. After careful enquiry you learn of a history of physical and sexual abuse. Or perhaps the 85-year-old woman before you has tears well in her eyes when discussing her children. You learn that, while there might be a picture of four in the photo, that she gave birth to five – her first was stillborn. Immediately, then, you can step up intervention to include evidence-based practices to deal with this new information.

In addition, there is an intention in the Life Story Interview model to step outside the client "frame" to engage an older adult so that more opportunities for dignity can be created along with increasing comfort in the experience of therapy and establishing firm foundations of trust. This approach is less formal than conventional clinical engagement where a client has self-referred, but the intention behind each question or phrase is no less therapeutic and can lead to more explicit work. Like Alvin Goldfarb's pioneering work in the 1950s where he came to suspect that seniors could benefit if they believed they were gaining mastery over the therapist – a supposed "protective parent" image –

(Steury and Blank 1977) so too do I believe that re-positioning the alliance without a focus on pathology or "problem issue" can be more fruitful. This undercover pre-therapy therapy is, I believe, the missing jigsaw piece to effectively engaging an older adult. After this stage, as alluded to earlier, explorations which foster a fuller or richer account of identity can be explored.

PERSONAL REFLECTION

1. What do you think about undercover pre-therapy therapy?

_____

_____

2. Did you agree that the second "Lucy example" was likely to bear more therapeutic fruit than the first? If not, why?

_____

_____

3. What aspect of the initial engagement process might you find hardest?

_____

_____

4. What aspect of the initial engagement process might you find easiest?

_____

_____

5. What has attracted you into working with seniors?

_____

_____

TYPES OF ENGAGEMENT

If you work from a multi-modal perspective then the selection of treatment modalities can be a little like wandering about a buffet – a bit of this and a scoop of that – so that eventually a certain combination meets the need of your client. That is what you hope for anyway. Even if you work strictly within a certain modality you will choose different responses according to the client's issues and goals. In Cognitive Behavioural Therapy you might choose an arousal reduction intervention for tension, graded activities for low mood and graded exposure for anxiety. A Narrative Therapist will have a keen eye out for any exceptions if the dominant story is overwhelming, or work with the client to externalize the problem if self-blame features. A Body Inclusive Trauma Therapist, informed by developments in neuropsychiatry and attachment research, would be particularly attuned to levels of arousal in the body. Their line of enquiry might vary depending on whether they notice high levels of tension or low energy states. Acceptance and Commitment Therapists are likely to use "creative hopelessness", which aims to disentangle clients from emotional control and avoidance and encourages them, instead, to be open to and observe the emotional experience. Different issues or therapist orientation can mean a different intervention slant. There is a smorgasbord of responses in any one evidence-based practice, depending on the issue, and there is an even greater array of therapy options other than those just mentioned. If this were a psychological theory buffet your eyes would be bulging with the choice! However, in this chapter I will only present you with a sample of issues and interventions that I find most salient or relevant. So instead of getting indigestion, I hope that you will feel pleasantly satiated.

Issue-specific interventions

The issues that I find most common in working psychotherapeutically with older people in care include the following: grief and loss, readiness to die, experiences of pain or stress, complex childhood trauma and experiences of post-traumatic stress. This is not an exhaustive list, or a sample of issues exclusive to an ageing population, but these issues continue to be thematic in my work.

Grief and loss

She sits over by her window. Her 94-year-old face is predictably creased with age but there is a vitality in how she speaks – vitality marred with pain. The kitchen clock nearby sends a soothing rhythm and the canaries under the pagoda trill a beautiful song. The sounds around are as varied as Mrs Fortune's story in their pitch, tone and mood. There are melodies of love and ability, and deeper notes of heartbreak and despair.

How she misses her husband Walter and little dog Miffy. How proud she is about completing a university degree at 70 (!) but how hard it is to find intellectually stimulating conversations with anyone, let alone her peers. She works the Internet but craves one to one. She has interest groups but hearing loss gets in the way and her bad knee makes it difficult for her to drive. Her outlook is more like one 20 years her junior – stuck inside a frail body and a mind that is feeling foggy with age. There is not just one loss, but many. Not grief just related to death but of many "deaths" or losses related to change. Her independent living unit is neat and her family support her but you can see the ache of her constriction.

She tells you how she saw the psychologist based at her doctor's surgery. "I couldn't really understand her," she shares, with a guilty look, "I only went twice." You wonder how this intelligent woman could not understand anyone but you also consider how those of the "lucky generation" might not easily engage with a therapist who is focusing too much on pathology and not adapting their techniques to be senior friendly, like a psychologist might with specialist training.

Sessions are a patchwork of structure and letting Mrs Fortune tell her story – intervention that has purpose but not in a way that interrupts a natural flow and the expression of feeling. It is a strategic dance between intuition and drawing on the evidence base – the art and science of good clinical practice. You look at photos (of Walter and Miffy) and ask her what she misses most. You listen patiently as she chokes with emotion when surveying a handout on experiences of grief[14] and identifying the ones relevant to her; as well sharing her responses to the "dual process model".[15] You learn about other losses she has experienced in the past and how she responded – what worked the best. You discover how Walter was pivotal in providing her with emotional strength in difficult times and was her intellectual peer. You ask about the context of his death and if she had a chance to say goodbye. "Are there any remaining things that you wished you could've said to him?" you wonder out loud.

Other questions include asking her what words of comfort Walter might give to her if he was with us now. Is there a special object that reminds her of him? How might she prepare for the "first" Christmas, his birthday, the anniversary of his death? You kindly explain how normal it is to talk to photos and wonder out loud how else she tries to maintain connection with her beloved. You are alert to serious intentions to join Walter but can see that, with each session, a burden appears to be lifting. You let her speak about what is most relevant and guide her in an exploration of meaning.

When you review therapy with her at session six Mrs Fortune says with appreciation, "I feel like I can talk to you. I still miss Walter terribly you know. But it doesn't feel as heavy [she places a hand over her heart]. I'm glad I got referred to you." You feel fortunate too – for being allowed to walk with this charming woman in her grief. "Sometimes I feel as if he is here with us," she says suddenly, then her mouth widens into a grin, "But not in a strange way." It is nice to see her smile.

No matter how positive you want to be, it is hard not to link "age with loss" like they are identical twins. Even though people of all ages can experience loss related to change, the fact is that older adults are often facing a level of loss unprecedented in their lives. And while not everyone interprets the same event in the same way – experiences a negative outcome – research indicates that relationship loss (not to mention other losses) increases the likelihood of mental illness developing (Baker and Procter 2015). Not only was Mrs Fortune grieving the loss of her husband and cherished dog, but also all manner of issues ranging from reduced physical capacity to increased social isolation.

Grief therapy, therefore, is all the more relevant for this population and the multiple layers of grief and loss can make it "complicated" (Kessler 2015). Mrs Fortune's grief was already complicated by virtue of the number of losses due to death and change. But complications could have also resulted if Walter's death was traumatic and witnessed by Mrs Fortune, if old losses (such as the death of a child) were triggered or other memories (perhaps related to war), if emotional expression was punished by punitive parents or teachers, if Mrs Fortune had been too dependent on her husband, or if their marriage had been infused with tension or abuse. Sometimes therapy can look a lot like peeling away the layers of an onion – once one layer is dealt with, another emerges.

For Mrs Fortune, an exploration of grief over her husband also brought to light many other experiences; a combination of primary, secondary and tertiary losses. For example, with her husband no longer alive, she has lost the regularity of someone to talk to and the status of being in a couple relationship (a secondary social loss). Such a loss also caused her mood to take a nose dive (tertiary loss) which challenged her usual self-image as someone who can cope with life's adversities. And while her husband's death would have resulted in condolences and ceremony, other losses might not be so acknowledged. The death of her little dog Miffy for instance, which happened two months after Walter died, did not attract a wake – but was felt almost as keenly.

And what of declining health? In Chapter 3 we reviewed the five interrelated types of senior distress: physical, neurological, social or spiritual, psychological, and environmental or lifestyle. In Mrs Fortune's case this might be translated into reduced vision, mobility and independence. But she might have felt uncomfortable seeing such loss as worth commenting on and think, "Well, what do you expect at my age?" We will look specifically at invitations to downplay late life distress in Chapter 8 but suffice to say here that these losses related to change can go unseen, be unacknowledged and make grief even more complicated, making it "disenfranchised grief" (Doka 1989, cited in Backhouse and Graham 2013; Misrachi 2012).

So, how do you process the death of someone or other losses? For decades the "gold standard" seen by many has been the stages model identified by Elizabeth Kübler-Ross in her 1969 book *On Death and Dying* – denial, anger, bargaining, depression, acceptance – where healing is progressive and reliant on successful navigation of each stage. But Hall (2011) and Misrachi (2015) have challenged this model, and ones like it, pointing to a lack of evidence to support its effectiveness. I agree. A client might look sheepishly at me: "I just can't get over it yet, you know, get to that acceptance stage." They seem to be wrestling between a desired state based on stage theory and a determination not to let a lifelong love dissolve into nothingness. This tension and guilt can lead to even greater distress.

The director of the Australian Centre for Grief and Bereavement, Christopher Hall, speaks about how the winds of change are affecting attitudes held in clinical psychology about stage theory. He writes:

> Long-held views about the grief experience have been discarded, with research evidence failing to support popular notions which construe grief as the navigation of a predictable emotional trajectory, leading from distress to "recovery". We have also witnessed a shift away from the idea that successful grieving requires "letting go" of the deceased, and a move towards a recognition of the potentially healthy role of maintaining continued bonds with the deceased. Recent research evidence has also failed to support popular notions that grieving is necessarily associated with depression, anxiety and PTSD or that a complex process of "working through" or engagement with "grief work" is critical to recovery. The absence of grief is no longer seen, by definition, as pathological. (Hall 2011, p.1)

Hall (2011) goes on to explain that there can be some merit in phase theory, so long as it encourages a dynamic and subtle understanding of experience:

The early stage theories of grief became unpopular because they were considered to be too rigid. There are, however, new models that succeed in identifying definite patterns and relations in the complex and idiosyncratic grief experience... These models serve both counsellors and clients by offering frameworks that guide interventions and enhance clients' self-awareness and self-efficacy. (p.2)

Hall (2011) emphasizes the "four tasks of mourning" by William Worden as one such theory:

Worden (2008) suggests that grieving should be considered as an active process that involves engagement with four tasks: (1) to accept the reality of the loss; (2) to process the pain of grief; (3) to adjust to a world without the deceased (including both internal, external and spiritual adjustments); and (4) to find an enduring connection with the deceased in the midst of embarking on a new life. (p.3)

This interest in finding an "enduring connection" appears to be similar to what White (1998) was referring to in his landmark piece "Saying 'Hullo' Again: The Incorporation of the Lost Relationship in the Resolution of Grief". For Mrs Fortune, this would mean instead of seeking closure, the therapist would encourage connection and acknowledge the enduring qualities of relationship even though a life has ended. In this way she might be more able to reconstruct meaning – a fundamental objective according to Neimeyer (2000) and supported by Hall (2011) – which can help people make sense of their lived experiences in a way that is important to them and that honours significant people in their life. But what appears absent in much of the literature around grief, still, is how it can relate to multiple loss late in life. Perhaps in time this will change if an ageing population become more vocal about what it is like to experience a tsunami of change.

Readiness to die

As a general rule, our Western society is not that comfortable talking about death (Kornfield 2008). Couple this with the principal goal in any health system being to preserve life then, understandably, talk about death can elicit a good deal of anxiety. Doctors may fear that they have failed their patient if they are not doing medical "back flips" to avoid death and decline and mental health professionals are mandated to detect and intervene if there is a threat to life. Everyone appears concerned with "managing risk" to maximize wellbeing – whether this is more about a fear of litigation or an interest to be beneficent will depend on the context and your point of view.

Desire to die statements are taken seriously. Health professionals working with people who have a life-limiting illness are encouraged to be active in engaging a patient wishing to die by asking, "Can you tell me why you wish your life to end?" or reinforcing that while they cannot legally assist them to die that they will do all in their power to help them be pain free (Hudson *et al.* 2006, p.708). However, there is debate about how much palliative care should aim for a "pain-free" death, citing an interest instead to use rating scales for clients to indicate how much pain they are in and how much pain would be all right for them to experience when dying (Whyte, personal communication, June 2017).

While the practice of euthanasia continues to be an ethical "hot potato", the fact is that most locations on the planet do not endorse the facilitation of death. This is for good reason, especially when it comes to older adults. Depression or feeling like a burden can cloud the judgement of an advanced senior, have them feeling like they have no control or choice and have them thinking that death is better than life (Hitchcock 2015). Believing in the sanctity of life and aiming to improve quality of life – at any age – is surely the stuff that health professionals should be made of: to help and "do no harm".

But with an interest in life can come a discomfort with death. Where are the opportunities to explore how someone *feels* about death? It is intriguing that, in the best practice guidelines for a palliative approach in working with older adults in the community, nowhere is death mentioned other than in relation to advanced care planning – it is not even in the section on psychosocial needs (Commonwealth of Australia 2011b). Books like *Dying to Know: Bringing Death to Life* facilitate a more emotional and philosophical exploration. Comments like, "People study for weeks for a birth. Why not study for a death?" and advice suggesting that, "It's quite normal to speak with the dead" (Pilotlight Australia 2007) in conjunction with poignant images encourage thought-provoking responses to a topic that many do not like to speak about or, as the following suggests, even think about.

My previous co-worker, who I mentioned earlier in Chapter 5, was once called out to see a lady in a facility who was threatening starvation.

While everyone seemed to be running around in panic that this lady was determined to die, my colleague did not buy into the angst or pressures to "fix" this woman. Instead, she offered her a wonderful opportunity to talk about why death was so important to her and what she hoped her life stood for. In the end, she was asked to disengage from delivering a service for fear that it might further fuel a desire to die. We did not know how things turned out for this lady but – whether she followed through with her wish or not – I am sure that my colleague's gentle and authentic interest was a ray of sunshine in her life.

The place between "desire to die" and "readiness to die" is like shades of grey. There can be a surprising array of variety in people's relationship with death at end of life. An interest in death could be about a sense of hopelessness, a resigned optimism about being free from suffering, an energetic determination to have control and choice, a calm acceptance of one's fate, contentment with a long life, irritation with being artificially preserved, or an active embracing of a spiritual context when death is drawing close. This section intentionally speaks of "readiness to die" as often this is overlooked or confused with suicidal ideation or intent, which was discussed in detail in Chapter 3 under "psychological distress". Many seniors want to live as long and as well as is humanly possible. But what of those who want to reflect on their life and think about death? What if you have lived a good life and you are just plain ready? Seniors do not usually have many years left so death, quite naturally, can be on their minds.

Psychotherapy can play a key role here because offering an open and confidential space to talk about hopes, fears and resentments at end of life can bring about much relief versus "holding it in" like you might your breath. It perhaps is worth mentioning here that it is not always helpful for family and friends to fill this role – either because of their own discomfort or because of how a senior might worry about the impact on their loved ones or fear their judgement. Every supportive relationship can have its place and, in the case of psychotherapy, it gives permission for clients to "get in and get dirty" like an invigorating dig in the garden on a bright sunny day.

Sometimes the senior will initiate conversations about death, sometimes we might need to. In both contexts a sense of choice and control can be promoted. Asking specific questions about how much information the senior wants to know if they are palliative can keep staff in step with what is important to that person. Maybe the resident wants to know every single detail; and maybe they do not and would prefer their significant other to be informed. If we do not ask then we might not know – and not asking can also lead to misunderstandings. To give an example, a geropsychologist once told me how she was asked to see a resident because staff were concerned that she had given up on life. This resident had stopped eating and was not getting out of bed. When my colleague came to see her she was expecting suicidal ideation. What she got instead was a surprise. Her resident had misunderstood. The form about "do not resuscitate" and "do not intubate" had been interpreted to mean that she was palliative. "No!" my colleague reassured her, "they are just routine questions for everyone." Satisfied that death was no longer imminent this lady reported to feel more relaxed, began eating again and started to engage in life once more. Equilibrium was restored once someone was brave enough to talk about the "d" word and what it had this person believing.

If you feel some avoidance toward issues related to death then, congratulations, you are human. As for aiming to preserve life, what could be more noble? It is just that when we have excessive fears about the topic of death, or become blinkered by our risk-averse priorities, then we are not able to create fruitful conversation spaces for those who are near death or who are ready to die or, as in the case above, are thinking that they are about to die when in fact they are not. Knight (2004) observes that many – especially young – therapists can feel quite anxious about discussing death with older adults and suggests that often it is "the therapist rather than the client who is fragile" (p.155). True.

So what can be done? I will refer to my geropsychologist colleague again. She suggests these tips: arrange to speak about death to someone close to you and who does not mind you "practising" on them, journal about your ideas on death, articulate your "worst nightmare" and your "best death", write your own fake obituary, or join a supervision group where other professionals are also working with death and the dying. Once you get over your own distress you can also revisit some misconceptions you might have. Are you thinking, like so many others do, that talking about death will only add to distress? If you have not already – I would invite you to try it. Talk about that "d" word with older adults. Some conversation openers could include:

- A lot of people find themselves thinking about death at your age. I was wondering if this is the case for you too?

- It can be hard, in a place like this, to be exposed to so much deterioration – people declining in health and dying. What's it been like for you living with this going on?

- Is it important for you to talk about any fears that you might have about death – or any wishes related to end of life?

- I was wondering how you feel at this "end of life point" in your life with death just around the corner?

- As you look back on your life and get closer to death, I was wondering what aspects of your life stand out as most significant? Ones that you would like to be remembered by?

Providing opportunities to explore issues related to end of life can create space for important past, present and future reflections, and a sense of value and fulfilment can be fostered right up until the very last breath. Instead of generating more angst you just might find the opposite – relief and peace. Is it not this that we would wish for someone near death?

Experiences of pain and stress

According to Goldberg and McGee (2011) on a United Kingdom based website biomedcentral.com, "Pain is an enormous problem globally" and warrants a public health response. Australia, as an example, is heeding this call and had a "campaign for pain" in 2016 which urged government to address pain as "one of the most neglected and misunderstood areas of healthcare" (Pain Australia 2017, p.3). Estimates are that "one in five Australians lives with chronic pain including adolescents and children. This prevalence rises to one in three people over the age of 65" (Blyth *et al.* 2001) and that the prevalence of chronic pain is projected to increase as Australia's population ages – from around 3.2 million in 2007 to 5 million by 2050 (MBF Foundation 2007). So chances are that if your caseload does not currently involve people experiencing chronic or persistent pain[16] – it soon will. And if you are already consulting advanced seniors who are living with persistent pain, then you are likely to see a whole lot more in time to come.

The Pain Australia website goes on to say that:

Older people and those living with a disability have the highest rates of chronic pain in our community. One in three people aged over 65 are living with chronic pain... In residential aged care, 92% of people are taking at least one analgesic medication daily and 80% of people report pain as a problem. (Pain Australia 2017b)

And with medication comes a compounding problem: side effects. Pain medication can worsen cognitive ability, create dizziness (increasing the risk of a fall) or negatively impact on a person's ability to concentrate. This is where you come in. If you have some experience in helping people manage distress then your skills can go a long way in helping seniors find non-medicinal relief from persistent pain. As the following will detail, there is strong support for non-medical interventions to help people cope with persistent pain. These interventions can also be generalized out to other experiences of distress as well. One non-medical treatment process for pain comes from Butler and Moseley's (2013) book *Explain Pain* which gained high praise in research and medical communities across the globe since its first release in 2003. The authors, with joint interests in physiotherapy and neurology, have also developed the Protectometer which allows patients to map and understand their pain story and devise individualized treatment plans (Moseley and Butler 2015). Central to the Protectometer is the concept of "danger pain" and knowledge based on neurological research which suggests that how we think and speak about pain affects the degree to which we experience it and how we behave as a result of this. If you are bracing yourself for the likelihood of pain then you are more likely to have heightened experiences of pain because your brain has become accustomed to over-protection and gets locked into an unhelpful arousal sequence.

Instead, the goal is to reverse such unhelpful processes by distinguishing between the evidence of danger and safety, speaking about pain in more neutral terms, being aware when you are in "the alert zone", and exploring how to experience pleasure in a body that also experiences pain. Another key element for their model includes the idea that effective treatment is based on the dynamic relationship between activity, beliefs/thoughts, previous experience of treatment, medications and psychosocial elements.

With research into neurobiology and neuroplasticity seeming to grow exponentially each day, there is now more acknowledgement of how powerful mind–body connections can be in either heightening or alleviating experiences of pain. Levine and Phillips (2013) suggest that "pain hypersensitivity" results when an over-active nervous system "goes rogue" (p.37). While pain in and of itself is not a bad thing as it can allow us to take good care of ourselves (Butler and Moseley 2013; O'Donoghue 2011), becoming overly frustrated, fearful or angry toward pain can worsen a person's situation. Meditation instructor and former psychotherapist Mark O'Donoghue calls this "secondary tension" and suggests that when this occurs, "…not only is there the primary pain, our reaction of dislike becomes a secondary pain. This sometimes takes the form of tightening around the primary injury" (O'Donoghue 2011, p.18). Meditations of loving-kindness[17] toward yourself can offset such an unhelpful response (O'Donoghue 2011) and "sitting with yourself in this practice [of loving-kindness] can be like sitting with a dear friend who is not well" (Levine and Phillips 2013).

Other meditation practices can also be helpful. Jon Kabat-Zinn (2013) was instrumental in fusing an East-meets-West model when he established the Mindfulness-Based Stress Reduction programme in 1979 to treat those with chronic experiences of pain and stress. Drawing primarily on Buddhist philosophy and practice, Kabat-Zinn (2013) emphasized the role of mindful breathing – non-judgemental focused attention in the present moment on the object of the breath – to help participants change the relationship they have with their body and experience one that is more helpful. This model then led to the development of Mindfulness-Based Cognitive Therapy (Segal, Williams and Teasdale 2002), which was initially used to prevent the relapse of depression.

Mindfulness skills are integral to a number of current evidence-based practices: Acceptance and Commitment Therapy, Mindfulness-Based Cognitive Therapy, Dialectical Behavioural Therapy, and Body Orientated Therapies for the treatment of trauma. The science of mindfulness can retrain the brain and change its very structure or chemistry through focused attention and repetition (Frallch 2012; Levine and Phillips 2013). Skills cultivated can include increased self-compassion, concentration, clarity, patience, wisdom, equanimity or stress tolerance, and an appreciation of changing states (Kabat-Zinn 2013; Kornfield 2008). But how can all this be used for an advanced senior? Here are some tips that might help:

- You are not likely to be able to use the "danger in me" (DIMS) and "safety in me" (SIMS) strategy on the Protectometer with them using sticky notes. They might not be able to read what you write for a start. But you could try and explain the general concept by clenching a fist indicating how habitual bracing for pain "just in case" could actually be more tiresome than judging events on a case by case basis and relating to them differently.

- Changing language around pain can often help defuse from the struggle with pain, moving instead to non-judgemental observation. For example, explore ways to discuss pain that sound less like they are speaking about a sworn enemy and more like a cool observation: the tingles, heat spikes, pulsations.

- If they start to look at you as if to say, "What would you know about pain and being my age?" then admit that you know nothing at all about what it is like for them. Resist any urge to spout the evidence base and, instead, suggest that they are way more qualified than you to judge if an intervention is effective or not and encourage open discussion around their experience of what you are working on together.

- Explore with them their pain story. Does it include unresolved emotional tension or trauma that might benefit from being attended to through supportive listening and self-regulation techniques (discussed in the next section)?

- Be alert for and highlight exceptions in their story – how has pain been successfully navigated in the past and what things do they currently enjoy despite also having experiences of pain?

- Provide an opportunity to grieve for a body that is no longer as comfortable and invite them to view their body with the tenderness of a mother to a crying baby.

- Encourage a simple practice where they imagine their breath going in and down to the pain-affected area and out through it – not aiming for reduced pain, but using the breath to care for their experience of discomfort and as a means to notice the difference between *thoughts* about the pain and the *actual changing states* of sensory experience.

Complex childhood trauma and PTSD

Trauma, just like persistent pain, can be eased considerably through learning how to regulate emotional and sensory experiences so that the limbic system[18] can settle (Levine and Phillips 2013). To illustrate this, I invite you to imagine your work with Mr Shoot. This English gentlemen is in his 90s living in long-term care and was referred to you by his GP who had diagnosed him with post-traumatic stress disorder (PTSD). He is a World War II veteran, having snuck in at age 17 and lied about his age, but trauma-related symptoms such as terrifying nightmares and flashbacks had only emerged in the last few years.

In the first visit you remember noticing a myriad of magnets on his fridge from his travels around Europe. This had him talking about his late wife who died six years ago. He missed her and had fond memories of their adventures in retirement. Other family memories were not so fond. His first wife was not good to him and his parents – this became an "access denied" zone. He let you ask more about his holidays though. He relaxed when he was talking about this and agreed for you to come back.

He was alert with a sweet smile and sat in his comfy chair with a walker by his side. For the next few sessions there was laughter, but you suspected that it was more a means to joke away the discomfort of why you were there.

"Don't know really what you can do for me," he said finally when discussion had centred on the idea of therapy. He had shrugged with resignation and said with eerie brightness, "This is my lot!" Was he trying to shoo you away? Would he try it and see, you had asked. "Oooh, I'm not sure," he had replied. Then, a story about last year's Remembrance Day service at the facility came out. He had never been to one in his life but staff had been so encouraging. He relented. "Bloody ended up crying like a baby. Stupid. I had to have two staff walk me back to my room!" He had laughed, but then looked at you like shame and fear were about to squeeze you out the door.

The next three sessions were like a push-pull dance about the idea of therapy. You got closer when you asked about the worst that could happen – crying, losing complete control – which allowed you to speak about how maintaining his comfort and control could feature in your work with him. It made sense. You remember the words of Babette Rothschild (2000) coming to mind, "First, do no harm" (p.77). She warned against the risk of re-traumatization and the value of slowly relieving the pressure, a little "pft" at a time, as if you were to safely lift the lid of a pressure cooker so it did not explode (Rothschild 2000, p.79). Mr Shoot did not want another explosion like Remembrance Day. He was done with that. You praised his intuitive ability to look after himself.

You remember feeling eternally thankful that most of your work to date had been able to be accomplished "undercover" – he would have run a mile otherwise. You also felt relieved that there were no session limits for, in trauma, more harm could be done with a short time frame (Kezelman and Stavropoulos 2012). Mr Shoot was still highly sceptical but admitted that, so far, things had been okay and he felt safe with you. He was reassured that therapy could happen without him even mentioning his war days. You worked with him collaboratively deciding on what to aim for: a few skills in present moment awareness, especially when having a flashback. There were also other agreements: being realistic about the unlikely possibility of getting rid of the nightmares because of not being able to consciously intervene when experiencing them, and agreeing that he did not need to talk about his war days if he did not want to. Finally, at session seven, you get the green light.

Session 8

"That's right, you can close your eyes if you want," you say, guiding Mr Shoot in a mindfulness session. The room feels peaceful and all is well. Suddenly, Mr Shoot speaks. "The roast was good yesterday. I think it's chicken for lunch today." You look up startled and patiently go over the instructions again. Well, you console yourself, at least he is becoming attuned to the state of his stomach! Focus on "the anchor"[19] activity resumes. "Now, I invite you to notice, even more, the sensations in your feet –" You are distracted by what you see as you glance up (first timers need monitoring). "Is something the matter?" you ask, seeing his furrowed brow. "I'm back there; the blood," he says simply. Oh. This isn't meant to happen. You realize your mistake and ensure that, from now on, he keeps his eyes open gazing at a spot in front. A debriefing session helps you iron out a few more issues but, overall, you are pleased that Mr Shoot was able to commit himself as best as he could to this short 5–10-minute activity. He agrees to practise it with you each time you meet.

Session 12

"I was sitting on my walker out on the street and suddenly all the cars became army tanks." Mr Shoot is describing a flashback. "What happened next?" you ask. You listen, elated, as you hear how Mr Shoot tried referencing his breath and "the anchor" activity. Concerns about him just trying to impress you waft away as, in his mind, he was still a failure for experiencing these intrusive hallucinations. But when you explain the importance of recovery he relaxes a little. "Well, I still don't like them," he concludes and you empathize while reminding him that the aim is not to be free of them – just learn how to recover from them.

Session 16

Your mouth is agape as you listen to Mr Shoot explain that he wants to talk about his war days. Okay, you think, but gradually. You jointly agree on setting a time limit – 10 minutes and then stop regardless to debrief and practise recovery skills before (during if needed) and after. You go through other safety procedures, "applying the brakes" as Rothschild (2000) says, by finding "safe" topics like his second wife and a facility carer called John whom he likes.

Session 19

Mr Shoot is talking a lot more freely now about the atrocities he witnessed. Both you and he are also feeling more confident in balancing effort with ease – delving down then coming back up (either naturally or intentionally) – so that his sense of control remains intact. Along with the trauma of war and a family history of neglect are softer storylines of mateship and longing. Through this you tap into his values – what things about his life and himself he has not wavered on – and when he weeps (yes, this is no longer so feared) you wonder out loud how this is honouring a mate's memory.

Session 21

At the previous session you had arrived to learn that Mr Shoot was in hospital with pneumonia. Today you find him with a breathing pump and fits of coughing. "But," he says valiantly through much coughing, "I think you've cured me!" Torn between curiosity and concern you wait for another round of coughing to subside. "I haven't had a nightmare for about three weeks." You realize, sheepishly, that you had forgotten to ask about this initial symptom, so captivated you had become with how he was finally finding a home for his story – and feeling at peace with his past. You both marvel at this progression but hasten to warn against any sense of failure should they return. You take this opportunity to review his experience with flashbacks. His face frowns deep in thought. He tells you that he can't remember when he last had one. Conversation returns to the past and he resumes talk about his mates, especially Thomas, and also his job when he returned from service.

Session 23

Mr Shoot is very ill today. He is too sick for a session. Staff know of his condition and he signals for you to sit down all the same, coughing profusely as he points to the chair. He takes your hand. You know touch is easier for him now than talking, and you just sit with him like this for a few moments. Then, through all the physical contortions, his weary eyes suddenly lighten. "Thank you," he says and stumbles through another round of coughing. Two days later and you get a message from the facility: Mr Shoot died peacefully in his sleep.

Trauma-informed care is about providing safety, trustworthiness, choice, collaboration, and empowerment (Kezelman and Stavropoulos 2012, p.10). For older adults trauma – complex childhood and/or post-traumatic stress disorder – can surface late in life even if they have been symptom free for decades (Daily Mail Australia 2012) which is likely due to age-related cognitive changes in memory and attention (Floyd, Rice and Black 2002). It is as if with age, extra time to reflect, and triggering events such as a disturbing news item, the "skin" that kept everything contained starts to get more thin and translucent (Tonkin, personal communication 2013) making it harder to keep down the demons of the past.

Mr Shoot's story is an example of how building trust is fundamental in trauma work with older adults and is a necessary foundation for supporting them to build a more stable relationship with their bodies and improve their regulatory capacity. It is also an example of work that is body orientated in that it addresses the sympathetic nervous system and is interested in neural integration. The evidence base for body orientated work in the treatment of trauma is building fast and this "bottom-up" approach cites the limitations of an exclusive "top-down" talking approach, such as in Cognitive Behavioural Therapy, because of how much these traditional models rely on conscious and explicit processes and can overlook somatic or implicit work focused on affect regulation – to the point of causing re-traumatization (Kezelman and Stavropoulos 2012, p.67). Pat Ogden (2012), founder of Sensorimotor Psychotherapy, explains this further by saying:

> A therapist's exclusive reliance on the "talking cure" to resolve symptoms of trauma and address implicit processing dynamics can limit clinical efficacy, because forming a coherent verbal narrative of past trauma is typically problematic. Traumatic memories are often not explicitly encoded (p.1)… A paradigm shift is indicated that privileges mindful awareness of the moment-by-moment *experience* of

implicit patterns over formulating a cohesive narrative, engaging in conversation, or "talking about". (p.2)

Ogden (2012, p.3) goes on to assert the need for a "dual focus" in body-orientated work: following the client's narrative while at the same time using mindfulness skills to be alert and curious to any implicit indication of unresolved trauma and looking for opportunities to build self-regulatory resources. With Mr Shoot this meant the following:

1. Noticing and responding to non-verbal indications of distress or dysregulated arousal, such as when he had started frowning when closing his eyes in a mindfulness activity and encouraging him to speak to his present moment experience. This can also be encouraged with comments that notice subtle changes in posture, breath, tone and movement such as, "Oh, your shoulders seem to bunch up as you talk about that" and "How are you feeling inside just now?"

2. A "dual focus" was used for safe trauma processing by allowing part of Mr Shoot's consciousness to connect with memories while keeping part of his consciousness connected to the therapist and the present moment.

3. Intentionally using the therapeutic alliance, through being mindful of both the therapist and the client's internal and external experiences, to build trust and relational safety. This process of connection and relationship development facilitates affect regulation and promotes trauma management in and of itself (Schore 2012).

4. Teaching Mr Shoot simple mindfulness-based strategies to help him develop strong connections with the present moment and create a distinction between the present moment and past memories.

5. Ensuring that Mr Shoot did not become overwhelmed and risk re-traumatization by discussion of traumatic experience if somatic distress was noted and shift to "safe topics" such as pleasant past memories or current interests, by encouraging him to compassionately relate to internal distress, and by containing or limiting the time allowed for verbal memory recall.

By adhering to the best practice standard clinical guideline of a three-phased approach – safety/stabilization, trauma processing, then integration (Kezelman and Stavropoulos 2012, p.7) – it appears as though there was a profound shift in Mr Shoot's brain where new neural pathways were formed and the "window of tolerance" (Siegel 2010, p.137) widened to expand his capacity to be receptive and experience equilibrium versus reactive in the face of stressors. By patiently tailoring interventions with ability and need, just sometimes, you can get more healing than anyone could have ever hoped for.[20]

Multimodal interventions

If you spend even just 40 minutes with an advanced senior aiming to intervene therapeutically you will probably notice how different it feels than work with younger populations. For one thing, if you are used to requesting that a number of forms be filled out either in session or between sessions – homework exercises – then you might need to let go of this expectation for a population who often struggle with writing, sight, memory, attention and energy. Not to mention a different style of investment in the therapy process – one that was probably not born of an expectation to get their psychological distress seen to. For intervention to be relevant, mainstream therapies need to be adjusted and therapy options that might not have evidence packed to the rafters should be considered.

Your ability to intervene using a particular modality *might* stretch out wide at times and look like work with those younger than 65. However, you will probably find that the range of talking therapy options will be limited according to the context and, if it were an elastic band like I mentioned in Chapter 4, it might look a little contracted. This can be frustrating and in the next chapter we will discuss this in more detail. However, the key point here is aiming to observe the nuances of your particular client and intervene accordingly (Wells *et al.* 2014). For seniors, the saying "fit the therapy to the person not the person to the therapy" is never more relevant.

The following will profile five modalities that I have found useful in my work with seniors: Acceptance and Commitment Therapy and Mindfulness-Based Interventions, Cognitive Behavioural Therapy, Interpersonal Therapy, Narrative Therapy, and Reminiscence Therapy. While there are a range of strategies that can promote emotional wellbeing in older people – physical activity, relaxation, sensory stimulation, music and arts, social activities, reflection, education and skills training, interventions that rely on technology, quality of life approaches, and interventions delivered by mental health professionals (Wells *et al.* 2014, pp.16–18) – it is this last category which relates to the talking therapies, about which, while information about clinical intervention abounds in the field of geropsychology, there appears to be little guidance from a mental health social worker practice informed viewpoint. Below is an attempt to provide such guidance, and for learning purposes, I will overview each modality as a discreet unit (in reality such interventions usually intertwine). To do this, I would like you to remember Harold whom you met in the introduction in "A special breed of senior". Do you recall how he has lost one leg, stays mostly in bed, has a wife called Elizabeth, and scored high for depressive symptoms? The following assumes that you have seen Harold for a number of sessions now. Imagine how you might intervene using each different modality:

Acceptance and Commitment Therapy (ACT) and mindfulness-based interventions

As you turn the corner into Harold's room you are surprised to see him sitting in his wheelchair. You have suggested this to him before but he had complained about the effort it took for staff to get him organized. He answers your raised eyebrow with, "Well, I can't just wither away in there," and looks at the bed. You agree and feel chuffed. There are other signs that Harold is engaging more in life and being responsive to his world. The curtains that once were drawn, strangling out the light, have been flung open these last few sessions at your urging. Today there is also a gentle breeze blowing which brings with it the smell of blossom. Perhaps, you think, it is time to go deeper.

If you were with a younger client you might already be "dancing around the hexaflex" having demonstrated "the struggle" and filled out a "bull's eye" sheet for values.

You might have even spoken about creative hopelessness. Your client could already have practised defusion techniques, connected with their present moment, learnt how to observe all types of thought content and begun talking about what they want to commit themselves to. With Harold, however, many of these things would be too abstract or effortful for his situation. Instead, you reach into your bag and get your values cards. You give him only seven at a time. "Just pick one in each group that you relate to the most. Our values can represent who we are – those things that have always been important to us and can still be even if we are in really different circumstances. Values are who we are inside – no matter what." He chooses ten overall, "belonging" being the one that speaks to him the most.

At another time you help him "notice five things" of what he can see, hear and feel. This has helped other residents you have seen to have a wide appreciation of their experience – not just what's going on in their head – but for Harold it only amplifies the reality of where he is and how ravaged his body is with discomfort. You try another tack. At your suggestion he identifies a painful emotion related to his situation and where he feels it most in his body. "Is it okay if we try something a bit different today? You can stop at any time if something doesn't feel right. This exercise is called BOLD. It stands for breathe, observe and open up to, listen and decide." With eyes closed Harold places his hand on where he feels distress the most. He learns that he can be bigger than painful emotions; that he does not have to get rid of them, but he can learn to breathe with them, and around them while bringing a sense of compassion to his experience. Later you are able to generalize this technique out to his physical pain.

With Mr Shoot in the previous section, mindfulness-based interventions helped with sensory integration and emotion regulation. For body-orientated therapies related to trauma or anxiety the role of mindfulness can go even deeper and encourage a dialogue of changing sensory experiences – located strongly in the present even if accessing a memory of the past.

For Harold, mindfulness strategies in the BOLD exercise encouraged an openness to unpleasant experiences related to the depressed mood. The breath remained the key object of awareness even while distress was contemplated. Demonstrating the futility of fighting unwelcome thoughts or experiences can still be done by grabbing your diary and placing it in front of your eyes, to show how much being caught up with thoughts can block your vision and deplete you of your energy. The alternative is to allow for the thoughts and feelings and this can be demonstrated by laying the diary on your lap. I just recommend that you do not do this in conjunction with the client as is usually encouraged (you are likely to be a lot stronger than an 88-year-old).

In using acceptance or mindfulness-based strategies you may not find yourself asking a resident to repeat, "lemons, lemons, lemons, lemons…" – an exercise to demonstrate the power of defusion – without them really writing you off! Understanding relational frame theory and the way that language can lock people into unworkable situations, an underpinning concept in ACT (Harris 2009), may not be realized fully with your senior clientele. But what you may be able to impart to them is a different way of relating to their experiences – one that is more compassionate and kind, and allows for an open embrace of emotions in the pursuit of valued living.

For those unfamiliar with ACT, the main objective is to promote psychological flexibility with clients by referring to the "hexaflex" – a model consisting of six interchangeable concepts and practices: present moment awareness, acceptance, cognitive defusion, observer self, connecting to values, and committed action (Harris 2009). In more simple terms the approach suggests that healing and wellness are achieved when people are present, open up to unpleasant experiences and do what matters, all the while adapting responses depending on workability (Harris 2009, p.13). Experience of psychopathology is suggested to relate to the opposite: psychological inflexibility as a result of living a conceptualized past and future without being instructed by the present moment, experiential avoidance, cognitive fusion, attachment to a conceptualized self, a lack of values and unworkable action (Harris 2009, p.27).

While debate continues as to whether "third wave" interventions such as ACT actually *replace* Cognitive Behavioural Therapy (CBT) or are just an *evolution* of it (Hofmann and Asmundson 2008), there appears to be a fundamental philosophical difference between the way ACT and CBT intervene with thoughts, which has implications for practice for any population. For example, the focus of CBT is to challenge or replace unhelpful thoughts. However, ACT techniques often centre around the practice of defusing from and accepting unhelpful thoughts. Therefore it is worth mentioning at this point that these different techniques – correction versus acceptance – would be confusing for a client if used in conjunction with each other. While the "committed action" component of the hexaflex can accommodate a variety of other interventions such as CBT, the stance on defusion is not consistent with a CBT approach. Overall, the evidence base for ACT is growing at a rapid rate and there is an appreciation of how it complements the "kit bag" for clinical psychology (Arch and Craske 2008; Heimberg and Ritter 2008).

Cognitive Behavioural Therapy

Your insistence to modify Harold's environment to include more natural light, in the early stages when Harold was least receptive to talking therapy, has paid off. So too has the gentle encouragement to appraise the minutest accomplishment – eating another mouthful of food – as an achievement without any expectation of enjoyment. A few sessions back you also did some problem-solving and relaxation work. He had been reluctant to go through the routine of getting out of bed based on earlier, and painful, experiences of staff not handling him sensitively enough. You had learnt about his needs, communicated them to staff, and practised with Harold how he could use imagery of a pleasant place to find reprieve when the process of getting changed and out of bed was at its worst. You also taught him some basic progressive muscle relaxation techniques which involved rotating attention to each main body part, tensing it if he could, then feeling the difference as it relaxed. This practice appeared to be particularly beneficial in the morning when Harold was anticipating his fears.

Today, you broach the idea of being more aware of how he thinks and the impact that this has on other experiences. "If it's okay with you we can look a bit more today about what's 'under the bonnet' up here [you point to your head]." Harold's face is a mixture of wariness and jest. "Don't know that there's much worth looking at there," he says. You proceed gently to explain that we are not failures for thinking all sorts of things but often what we think can be like getting caught up in a really unhealthy diet – how often addressing our "thought diet" and replacing it with better "food" can be really helpful. You wonder out loud what sorts of "food" he has been eating.

He begins to talk about the literal food of late, "Wouldn't feed that to a dog!" he laments. You empathize and press on realizing your need to be more concrete but still use Harold's candid reflections of nursing home cuisine to make your point. Using a visual aid you educate Harold about the thought-feel-sense-behave cycle and ask him if he can identify any unhelpful thoughts. He looks at you blankly. "I've heard you speak a lot lately about how hopeless you feel," you venture. "Might one thought be, 'I'm hopeless' or 'things are hopeless'?"

Harold agrees and you patiently explore how these thoughts have an impact elsewhere and create a spiral downward effect. "What about we try and interrupt that negative cycle?" you suggest and with Harold's consent you write a note in his therapy diary (for him and his wife Elizabeth) about being more aware of negative thoughts popping up, and how they create a chain of events for other aspects of his experience, such as the snowballing effect of low mood and how it can translate into not wanting to get out of bed – making him even more vulnerable to negative thought and mood patterns. You have already met with Elizabeth once and you were grateful how willing she sounded to consult your notes and support your work with Harold; she understood how this work requires a team approach.

For the next session, in Harold's example above, you would explore with him other more helpful cognitions like, "I'm not stupid just because I'm feeling sad," "I still have Elizabeth who visits me," "I am not like a baby if I cry," "I might not be able to walk but I can still talk to those I care about," "I miss not living at home but it is better on Elizabeth that I'm here and safer for me" and "I have survived hard times in the past." On this last point you could build on what you know already about the difficult experience of losing a daughter in an accident when she was 22 and the inner reserve he drew on to cope. Infusing a strength perspective can increase client confidence by locating past success (think of how much change these seniors have had to navigate!). Together, affirming strengths, challenging cognitive distortions,[21] finding evidence to support an alternative view, replacing unhelpful thought content with more helpful ones, and reinforcing change with reward all can work together to improve emotional and psychological wellbeing.

With Harold, you could also begin exposure work. Gradually Harold could stay out of bed longer, take one meal a week in the dining area – then three, try out the Lifestyle activity where he can play bowls in his wheelchair, visit home, see some friends at the bowling club. In this way you could infuse pleasant events scheduling with a progressive layering of difficulty, frequency and intensity. One word of warning however. Be sure to allow plenty of emotional validation before embarking on a rational process of change – otherwise reappraisal can turn into a grim request to "just look on the brighter side of life". All well and good for you to say.

Cognitive reappraisal and restructuring are core components of any Cognitive Behavioural Therapy (APS, OTA and AASW 2011). In the example above, Harold has begun to consider a different way of looking at simple daily activities and also the notion that what he thinks about himself and his situation can either help or hinder him. Whether CBT is more or less accessible and empowering for an older adult can depend on your viewpoint. For some the metacognitive – thinking about thoughts – element is helpful for a population who often have reduced capacity for abstraction because cognitive replacement suggestions like "I am not stupid just because I'm feeling sad" can be concrete. Furthermore, interventions that include repetitive practice, graded exposure, visual cues, psychoeducation and recording unhelpful thought patterns are seen by many as skills that lend themselves easily to being taught and reinforced. It can also be seen as empowering if your older adult clientele feel more comfortable with a directive style – such as what they might expect from a doctor. However, if you are of the opinion that thinking about thoughts is, in and of itself, an abstract endeavour not lending itself easily to cognitive decline then you might not see CBT as accessible for this clientele; not to mention that people like Harold are of a generation not used to psychological concepts. And if you believe that an older adult's comfort with having a professional tell them what they should do is just evidence of disempowerment then working purely from a traditional CBT model with this population might not be for you.

Interpersonal Therapy

"Hello Elizabeth," you say as you meet this neatly dressed woman for the second time. Her pearl earrings wobble as you shake her hand. She has welcoming hazel eyes and a complexion that is yielding to a lifetime enjoyment of the great outdoors. You could have used the doctor's room for this session – Harold is feeling more comfortable spending longer periods in his wheelchair and moving about – but you suspect that Harold's room has the familiarity that they need for this couple session.

It is easy referencing the importance of relationship to this loving couple. Conversation flows to exploring how individually and as a couple they have experienced grief and weathered hard times – together. There are fresh tears over their daughter Susan whose life was tragically cut short. Harold's current complicated grief is understood in terms of how he was socialized to suppress emotion when he was young, praised by his wife for being "strong" when Susan died, and feeling emasculated after hospitalization and no longer being able to perform the roles through which he found identity and meaning.

Elizabeth gets out a handkerchief and goes to wipe Harold's tear-stained face. "There we are darlin'. You'll be right. Just think of what a great father you were for Susan." You see your opportunity. "Yes Harold, I'm sure you were a great father to Susan. Her loss was an absolute tragedy." Turning to

Elizabeth you suggest, "Elizabeth, thank you for comforting Harold just now – you both obviously care for each other a lot. I was wondering, however [turning to Harold], how it felt with what Elizabeth did just now?" Quickly qualifying you add, "Sometimes well-meaning gestures happen out of habit or are simply a case of being unaware of other things that could be happening as a consequence. [looking at Harold] Would it have been easier, for example, if Elizabeth had not drawn attention to your tears or maybe encouraged them as she handed you the handkerchief?" Harold nods tentatively in agreement and you turn to Elizabeth.

"Elizabeth, what just happened now could be a wonderful opportunity for you both to learn how to support each other more at this difficult time. Is it okay if I just run a few other things past Harold?" Elizabeth nods and you sense that, while a little wary, enough trust has already been developed and you proceed to explore how Elizabeth might interact with Harold in ways that help ease embarrassment about releasing pent-up emotion and help promote independence.

Could she give him the handkerchief and let him attend to his needs himself? What other things could she let go of doing for Harold when he is capable of doing them on his own? Are there some simple jobs that she can allocate back to Harold – roles he used to perform like coordinating the weekly sweepstakes for their bowling club, and deciding which handyman is best for maintenance work on their apartment. After all, you muse out loud, she has enough on her plate already with the number of extra duties she has had to take on! This reflection sends the message you intend to – one of warmth and support. The relief on Elizabeth's face, the tremor of a chin, are signs that she indeed feels burdened by her current lot and, together, you work out how communication can maximize respect and wellbeing.

Being interpersonally sensitive is integral for the above work or any other type of family therapy. The Interpersonal Therapist seeks to direct change at the relationship level – to the four problem areas – grief, interpersonal role disputes, role transitions, and interpersonal sensitivities – as this is seen to either maintain or alleviate individual distress (Howell, Murphy and Opolski 2009, p.14). In time Harold's relationship with best friend Ralph, and his wider social network, could also be an avenue through which to address improved functioning. There are benefits and challenges of using Interpersonal Therapy (IPT) with an older adult population. The challenge is that the very fact of being an advanced senior – or oldest old – can mean a reduced pool of significant others. The issue might be less about interpersonal issues in their life than the fact that there are no significant ones or ones that they find meaningful and want to cultivate. However, an advantage with IPT for older adults is how easily it lends itself to issues common for this group, like role transitions, and the importance of strengthening whatever interpersonal networks are available to manage intrapersonal concerns related to change or decline. Finally, interpersonal issues can become more complex with age where there is greater reliance on adult children, involvement of proxies, and increased exposure to a multitude of staff and residents if needing to move into long-term care.

Narrative Therapy

"I should be over this now. It's stupid." Harold's face scrunches. "It's stupid" could well be translated to "I'm stupid." Noises are heard in the corridor. The voices of staff penetrate through the closed door. The voices in Harold's mind are more intrusive. "Has 'this stupid thing' been around just recently or has it got a long history?" In this one question there is a major shift. You and Harold are now no longer examining how he is the problem – how personally fused he is to his own distress – but how this problem exists in an external space outside of him. It is as if you are both looking at it together as equals. "Shame" is what it is eventually called after consulting with Harold on exactly the right terminology to describe this problem.

It turns out that "shame" has been around for a very long time. You learn about how Harold was often scolded by his father, especially if he cried, how he spent five years in boarding school and was mercilessly teased, and how Harold felt about having shame in his life. "I probably deserve it," he says one time. "Oh," you are surprised. "Could that be another one of its tactics do you think? Having you believe that you deserve it?" Harold looks a little puzzled, then thoughtful; "Yes," he says simply.

As he talks about his life with shame there are glimmers of exceptions – times when shame has not been so strong. Even times when it was not present at all. You are very interested in this and ask more about the conditions that made this possible. "I was wondering," you venture, "what inner resources you drew on to keep shame shut out like this?" Other questions you ask: Have other people noticed this ability in you to keep shame at bay? If they were here now what might they have said about the destructive effects of shame on you? How might they have felt about this? If there was one thing that they particularly admired about your efforts to keep clear of shame then what would that be? Did shame's presence always seem as if it were destructive or were there moments that it also contributed to Harold's life. Conversation returns to present-day concerns. How has shame tried to weasel its way in lately? Might Elizabeth have noticed this? What could happen if it continued to get its way? How did Harold feel about this? Gradually, Harold builds a position against shame and is encouraged to examine how it tries to work in his life and how he relates to it.

In many sessions, conversations about shame lead back to when his daughter Susan died. You encourage a couple session where Elizabeth is present and give them both an opportunity to honour the loss that was their daughter. Harold begins to berate himself while exploring his grief and there is a lighter moment when you observe how shame is being particularly flaunty today. Harold and Elizabeth laugh as you go on to describe how it might look if it were parading itself in the Christmas Pageant. Then the mood takes on a mellow tone again as you explore with them both how they can "say hullo again" to their cherished daughter instead of feeling like they have failed in their grief work. "After all these years," Harold says, "and it still gets me here [he points to his stomach]." Overall, Harold learns to actively position himself against shame and explore more fully what matters most to him and what that says about the sort of person he is. Shame sulks in the corner of his room while hope peers shyly around his door.

Narrative Therapy is being embraced as a clinically relevant practice in the field of gerontology because of how it explores the relationship people have with their life stories (Caldwell 2005; Moore *et al.* 2000). While the breadth of research on the efficacy of Narrative Therapy is continuing to expand generally, particularly in North America (Russell, personal communication, 2017), the evidence base in relation to older adults specifically has much room to grow (Wells *et al.* 2014). From a Narrative Therapy stance, positive change is brought about through an emphasis on personal agency, considerations of power, and meaning making as the therapist re-engages people with their life histories and explores with them their interests for the future (Dulwich Centre Publications 1999; Morgan 1999; White 2000, 2005; White and Epston 1989).

In the case of Harold it meant creating opportunities to examine the influence of various institutions (family/society) or dominant stories on his life , learn how "shame" developed in these contexts and limited positive self-definitions or healing. It also meant exploring values or identities that were important to him, drawing on the metaphor of connection – or saying hello again – to help Harold in his grief work with regard to his daughter Susan and co-authoring self-definitions that acknowledged Harold's ability to distance himself from "shame".

This process of co-authoring relies on the therapist to be "decentred and influential" (White 2005, p.9) and partake in deconstructing expert knowledges by viewing clients as the primary author of such knowledges and practices (White 1992). Therapists strive to keep the client "centre stage"; be decentred, by not imposing their own interpretations or agendas and by being responsive to information that emerges as important for the client. Therapists are also influential through a scaffolding process of reflection and questions that uncover hidden knowledges or skills in the client and – jointly with the client – develop rich understandings of how the client wants to live their lives. Stephen Gaddis (2014, p.1) adds an understanding of the "de-centred and influential" stance by explaining that:

From a narrative perspective, we must acknowledge that there is never any neutral place to stand when it comes to meaning making or story development. At every moment in relationship, we are either centering our own meanings or we are centering someone else's…we have an ever-present responsibility for how we engage with someone, even when they are at the center of meaning-making.

Through its consultative style and disinterest in the therapist assuming an expert position, this therapy can explicitly and implicitly foster deep respect and value for the unique views of the senior – their wishes, hopes and what they hold to be valuable – and trust in their ability to facilitate change.

Reminiscence Therapy or Life Review

Looking over at a photograph you suggest engaging in some Life Review work: "A chance to take stock of your life, review accomplishments, and not let your current circumstances steal from you the pleasant memories of your past. Maybe, even, there are some regrets or painful memories that need to be dealt with – but everything at your pace and only if you want. After all, 88 years is a lot of life that's been lived!" He does not argue with you on that one.

Elizabeth helps out by ensuring that a pile of photo albums are left to peruse over at your next session. Through semi-structured questions you talk about the parts of his life that he most wants to first. This begins in his early 20s when he met Elizabeth. Conversations after that dance pre and post this point – retirement, hard memories of childhood, adolescence, a lifetime of bowls, losing Susan, his friends – but all the while create space for meaningful reflections.

You are struck by how engaged he has become in this process. He says that these conversations are the highlight of his week. He appears to relish an opportunity to connect with important memories of the past and find relief for those issues left unresolved. This process also appears to strengthen for him a sense of identity. You wonder if this is the case for him and he agrees. He likes you suggesting that this identity

COUNSELLING AND PSYCHOTHERAPY WITH OLDER PEOPLE IN CARE

is his core self – a self that cannot be touched by age or illness or disability, that can remain protected in him always. It is as if he is becoming friends with himself again and you delight in facilitating this meet. You also note that when he is engaged in this process that he does not lament about his pain and discomfort as much. It is like he is transported to another place.

After many sessions, a large amount of information and numerous quotes are gathered. Some of this relates to factual elements about family and historical events – personal and on a world scale. And some of what you have relates to his interpretations and what has become relevant to him in the therapeutic process. He has a nephew who generously scans a number of photos and memorabilia. You also explore with him significant metaphorical images that you get from the internet and collaborate with him on short texts that could accompany each picture like: a bulldog hanging onto a rope with "I always manage to hang in there," a bowling green and carpet bowls with "I still love my bowls," a tear with "Sometimes I cry as we all do when we feel sad," a tombstone with "I have had hard times and...," a picture of a bright sunflower with "I've had good times."

All of this becomes a Life Journey Booklet – a picture story with simple text – which Lifestyle compile under your guidance. Elizabeth has plans to take some elements of the booklet and turn it into a DVD for Harold's ninetieth, complete with his favourite tunes. It is more than just a bibliographical account of his life. It embodies key elements of his identity, locates significant others, articulates an emotional experience, creates a meaningful exploration of his past, and reinforces strategies that he finds helpful to deal with the present. After you show him a draft version he sits in stunned appreciation. "Well now..." is all he can manage to say.

Because there is an evidence base for using reminiscence and Life Review therapies with older adults in community and facility settings (Caldwell 2005; Knight 2004; Wells *et al.* 2014), to view one's life with integrity versus despair as in the last stage of Erikson's psychosocial development theory, it is curious that it is not listed as a

Focused Psychological Strategy under Medicare in Australia. Perhaps, in time to come, it will be as a greater number of older adults seek psychological consultation and practitioners seek senior-friendly interventions – as is already the case in other parts of the world.

An integrated model for intervention

Have you ever been in front of a client and suddenly lost your way? You are not able to see the woods for all the trees of problems and you have a serious case of theoretical hyper-arousal – a deer in headlights. Or if you were dancing it might be akin to being so focused on the routine that you end up falling on the floor! Work with seniors can be like this. Often. The path you imagined going down has been hijacked, the co-morbidities are as numerous as the stars, and your client is looking at you like an exotic plant species – interesting but perhaps a little dangerous. In times like these you might need more than just a few Minties!

I have found that in times like these I need to lose my interest in the dance routine, and just move to the music. Connect. Be present. Work with advanced seniors, perhaps more than for any other group of adults, demands an ability to be present first and foremost. It is from this place that everything else can grow – dignity, respect, trust – and then deeper healing. But irrespective of anything else that you might do with them, what can be more beautiful than to gift them your interest in their story and your attention? I have had counselling students and colleagues ask me out of worry if they are doing enough. I believe that if you are truly present with your client and interested in them as a person then you are *always* doing enough. Period. Your skills and knowledge might add to that baseline in important ways but if you focus on connection then you are always doing enough.

This emphasis on human connection is not new. It can be found in the revolutionary work of Carl Rogers with his Human Potential Movement and concepts for psychotherapy such as being "person-centred" and having "unconditional positive regard". He also spoke about being real:

> I find it very satisfying when I can be real, when I can be close to whatever it is that is going on in within me. I like it when I can listen to myself... In place of the term "realness" I have sometimes used the

word "congruence". By this I mean that when my experiencing of this moment is present in my awareness and when what is present in my awareness is present in my communication, then each of these three levels matches or is congruent. ... I have learned...that realness, or genuineness, or congruence – whatever term you wish to give it – is a fundamental basis for the best of communication. (Rogers 1995, p.14)

I agree. And I believe that when I am connecting on a fundamentally human level in my work with older adults – holding this element higher than anything else I might have in my "clinician's toolbox" – then I have all I need to create constructive therapeutic encounters.

Work with seniors can be fascinatingly complex and unshakeably simple – all at once. It is complex because there are many things to consider as you take in all of the changing variables of environment, presentation, abilities and possible response pathways. But it is simple in that it can have, at its core, an emphasis on the therapeutic alliance and the pureness of being present in this moment with this person; in a way that penetrates beyond the shell of age or pathology and looks into the soul of the human.

As I have said before, I believe that there is an art and a science to this work. The therapeutic alliance or "realness" that you bring to your work could be considered an art – difficult to quantify and deconstruct in a way that is replicable. Then there is the science. The research-based confidence that tells us that certain interventions are likely to produce certain outcomes. But, as Allan Schore (2012) suggests in the title of his book, there is also *The Science of the Art of Psychotherapy*. He proposes the "regulation theory" (Schore 2012, p.2) for trauma management which is grounded in neuropsychiatry and attachment research. In this instance the spotlight falls fairly and squarely on the relational qualities of the therapist: their ability to develop a strong therapeutic alliance and be present to the internal and external experiences of, not only their client, but also themselves as they are counselling. Schore (2012) explains the principles and science for his theory:

We suggest that clinical expertise, especially with severely disturbed patients, relies more on nonconscious nonverbal right brain than conscious verbal left brain functions. Clinical efficacy is more than explicit left hemispheric technical skill in interpretation. Rather, increasing levels of clinical effectiveness with a broader spectrum of patients fundamentally involves more complex learning of a number of nonconscious functions of the therapist's right brain that are expressed in the therapeutic alliance. All technique sits atop these right brain implicit skills, which deepen and expand with clinical experience: the ability to receive and express nonverbal affective communications; clinical sensitivity; use of subjectivity/intersubjectivity; empathy; and affect regulation. (p.42)

If you think back to Mrs Need in Chapter 5 you might remember the proposition that therapeutic encounters were more likely to be fruitful if the therapist focused less on her pathology and more on her as a person, more on a foundational interest in connection than on formal engagement. This approach combines the "realness" that Rogers (1995) sought and the relational qualities that Schore (2012) argues are critical for effective psychotherapy. Connection with older adults in therapy is not just a building block for rapport; it is a foundational concept upon which everything else is built *and* it is a constant touchstone throughout each session and the course of therapy. To add some signposts to what I am suggesting, I have developed the following model (see Figure 6.1) that considers the breadth and depth of this dynamic interplay. The sections in black are considered "formal engagement" opportunities and the grey circle in the middle represents "informal or foundational engagement".

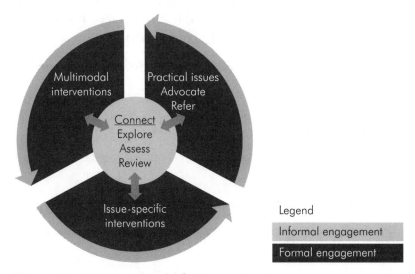

Figure 6.1: An integrated model for intervention

Formal engagement

All of these sections have been discussed in detail already. In Chapter 4 you learnt about the moving wheel of assessment. This mostly relates to the section in Figure 6.1 entitled "practical issues, advocate, refer". Yes, there is an element of assessment for informal engagement but primarily this model situates assessment in the realm of determining suitability and taking practical and explicit steps to alleviate suffering.

The last two sections on the outer circle relate to what has been discussed in this chapter: "issue-specific interventions" and "multi-modal interventions". As Figure 6.1 illustrates, intervention is not likely to stay in one particular area; it may rotate around *and* shift back and forth between the formal and informal domains. While it is more likely for therapy to be located in the informal domain at the beginning of contact and in the formal domain as contact continues, responding to need and circumstance means being able to move fluidly between both domains at *all* points and stages of contact.

Informal or foundational engagement

If you remember back to Chapter 5 where we looked at "invitations of engagement", you will be in a good position to learn more about informal engagement – a key feature of our integrated model for intervention. You will recall from this chapter that five guiding principles formed a bedrock for the initial contact phase:

1. *Dignity* How can you build them up? (Not in a patronizing or unauthentic way.)

2. *Choice* How can you help them feel like they are in control of the process?

3. *Value* What is it about their conversation that speaks of important values?

4. *Trust* What opportunities are there to reaffirm their trust in you?

5. *Permission to talk* How can you comfortably invite them into conversation?

The intention to connect and "just be", the primary focus of foundational engagement, is an embodiment of these principles. It also relates to the principles of "realness" mentioned earlier, developing a strong therapeutic alliance and using the mindfulness awareness that Ogden (2012) speaks about that is "integrated with and embedded within what transpires moment-to-moment between therapist and patient" (p.3).

You might also recall my suggestion in Chapter 5 to "free yourself from the cobwebs of agenda and just relax into your interest of this person as a human being". This is akin to forgetting about the dance routine for a while and just moving to the music. Yes, it might sound like an oxymoron to free yourself from an agenda and yet be alert to guiding principles. Perhaps it would help if the process of informal or foundational engagement is understood as having a *different* agenda to the one common in mainstream psychology? An agenda that is focused on the commonality of being human with all its struggles, rather than classification and diagnoses; and all the while using important "right brain" functions to build strong therapeutic alliances.

This change in emphasis is similar to the conceptual framework that McCormack (2003) developed when considering nursing practice with older people in the United Kingdom. He identified that the idea of a person-centred approach was already "embedded in the language of multidisciplinary practice with older people" (p.202) in his country but built on this by researching what autonomy meant for older people in hospital settings. McCormack (2003) was interested in thinking "beyond concepts of cure based on scientific facts and technical competence, to the adoption of a more holistic approach" (p.203). This is like leaving to one side the usual agenda of psychotherapeutic processes – mainstream psychology – and creating space for more informal engagement.

Moreover, McCormack (2003) strongly links the development of autonomy in older adults, desirable because of how independence is often under threat, with "authentic consciousness" that orientates nurses toward the personhood of the patient. Autonomy is suggested to be further strengthened when nurses engage in "imperfect duties" which are guiding principles like "compassion, concern, benevolence, respect and care" (p.204). Surely all these qualities already feature in a counselling interaction? Yes, our interest in a senior's wellbeing, our reflective listening skills, and our orientation toward hearing their story place us in a position to reduce suffering but how often is our agenda blinkered by a focus on symptomology, client goals, formal assessment and case conceptualization?

Being comfortable with an approach that includes informal engagement optimizes not only trust but also the choice that Dignity Therapy advocates for and the deep respect that is central to Narrative Therapy. When I first see advanced seniors they are not usually thinking in terms of therapeutic goals – or even of therapy. I remember explaining the process of counselling to one 95-year-old woman after informally engaging her and seeing the look on her face. I reflected back her scepticism. "What could talking do?" I asked rhetorically. "Exactly!" she exclaimed. But when I referenced the conversation we had just had she admitted to feeling very relieved. She was not able to articulate therapy goals but after an experiential understanding of counselling (via informal engagement) we were able to form them together: "You're interested in finding some more relief from your pain?" – "Yes," she replied. "To find a sense of peace about what your life has all been about?" I suggested – (teary) "Oh, yes."

Granted, psychotherapy may not be something sought by the people whom you first see on an informal basis, but by engaging in this way you can open the funnel of possibility wide and make the idea of therapy more palatable. And whenever you feel like you are at a stalemate, you can drop down into informal engagement so doubt or frustration can turn into relaxed curiosity. The senior before you becomes more a person than a client. The context becomes one where you are consulting them more than guiding them. A great way to do this is through the Life Story Interview discussed in Chapter 5. It is semi-structured and individualized in a way that Reminiscence Therapy is often not, and it can be free-flowing and clinically therapeutic in a way that Haight's (1982) Life Review and Experiencing Form was not designed to be.

While reminiscence, Life Review work and the interview process all create possibilities for seniors to access positive memories and/or deal with regret, only the Life Story Interview is an approach that can be used in all of the following ways: as an informal enquiry to develop knowledge and trust, as a segue into formal engagement, or as a formal process of therapeutic engagement that uses reminiscence work for reappraisal, accessing positive memories, strengthening identity and discovering meaning. The Life Story Interview, therefore, can help the therapist connect when in the informal domain, and can orientate a worker toward a relaxed interest in the senior's life – past or present. Informal or foundational engagement is, I believe, an essential ingredient for an integrated and effective way to work with seniors.

It is my opinion, and I expect that of many others, that intervention with seniors is more than just a formal process. However, this is not how clinical practice usually operates. Typical clinical transactions are often strongly framed by formal engagement processes: the client has referred themselves, the role of therapy and the therapist is explicit, the problem is the focus, the environment is usually a counselling room, and intervention leans toward a particular modality – usually an evidence-based practice – at any given time. Even geropsychologists speak about their initial contact as if they are honing in on symptomology and focused on developing an effective case conceptualization depending on whether presentation relates mainly to depression or anxiety. Is it possible that client dignity could be unwittingly compromised by engaging in this way? Is it also possible that this more formal approach makes therapy less accessible to the majority of advanced seniors for whom psychological intervention is as alien to them as a Martian is to an earthling? By having a model that incorporates both informal and formal engagement, therapy can become a process that is highly flexible and truly senior friendly.

To summarize, the issues salient to my work with seniors are: grief and coping with change and loss, readiness or desire to die, experiences of pain and complex childhood trauma or the presence of unresolved PTSD. While individual experiences will vary, it is important that therapists working with seniors have an understanding of these common issues and have basic competence in their ability to engage therapeutically in these areas. In addition, competence with a number of modalities is desirable as well as an ability to adapt these modalities to an advanced senior or co-morbidity context. But formally engaging in this way is only part of the picture. Equally important, especially in the first few interactions with a senior, is informal engagement which demands a suspension of practice that is framed tightly within the outcomes based medical model. All of this – exploring melancholy themes, adapting mainstream psychological practices, and responding flexibly to maximize engagement – can be very demanding. Challenges range from the overt to the subtle but surviving, and even thriving, in work with seniors is what the next chapter is all about.

PERSONAL REFLECTION

1. Which issue-specific intervention was most familiar to you and why?

_____

_____

2. Was there an issue that you felt least familiar or comfortable with? If so, you may want to reflect on this here.

_____

_____

3. What psychological modality do you lean most toward and why?

_____

_____

4. Which modality are you least interested in or comfortable with?

_____

_____

5. Do you have any reflections on the integrated model for intervention that was presented?

_____

_____

PART 3

THE BIGGER PICTURE

CHAPTER 7

CARING FOR YOU THE PSYCHOTHERAPIST

If you have been a psychotherapist for a number of years you would be used to the concept of looking after yourself. You have to. Your wellbeing and ability to listen to countless stories of distress depend on it. No doubt you already have a few tricks up your sleeve to tend to your energy levels and emotional needs. Maybe it is to release through social media, spend time in the garden, hang with your favourite friends, debrief with a colleague or supervisor, take a walk of solitude along the beach, become engrossed in a book, treasure time with family or say the dreaded "no" word. In big ways and small we try and balance all of our demands and keep our batteries charged. We know about burnout. We are alert to if we are feeling too exhausted, seeking a bit too much solace in that glass of red, becoming too emotional or irritable, or becoming affected by vicarious trauma. So what other issues are there to be alert to if you are working psychotherapeutically with seniors? Far from being an exhaustive list, the issues below are the product of my own experience and ones that may be helpful for you too.

The Mickey Mouse Mindset

"It was a bit 'Mickey Mouse'," your friend complains to you after returning from a beginners lesson on the ski slopes. They are an accomplished ice skater and will move up to the next level tomorrow so that they can get the extension they need. Mickey Mouse – it is a phrase that is a little derogatory or, at best, refers to something that is fairly basic. As you would guess by now, psychotherapy with seniors is far from basic and yet anything to do with working with older adults seems to bring with it an overly sweet affirmation, is dismissed outright, or met with veiled repulsion. Much of this, I suspect, is to do with society's general attitude toward ageing which is the subject of Chapter 8. But whatever the reason, identifying and dealing with the Mickey Mouse Mindset can be an important piece of armour to prevent you from becoming unnecessarily unsettled in your work.

I might meet a new worker, from another team, in the lunch room. When I mention that I work with older adults they go all gooey, "Ooh...," then laugh, "you must get lots of cups of tea!" Yes, I can see that image too. A quaint chat with somebody's grandma, sipping cups of tea and talking about the weather – oh, and a little bit about how they feel, maybe. This "down playing" can also be noted in the experience of other professionals working with older adults. For example, care managers and clinical nurses have lamented to me that amongst their peers they feel looked down on because they work in aged care. Furthermore, Doctor Karen Hitchcock (2015) in her explosive essay on caring for the elderly entitled "Dear Life", tells of the waft of disdain afforded to those who rub shoulders with the frail. She writes,

> My supervisor asked me, "Have you considered general medicine?"
> I had not.
> "Don't do it!" an endocrinologist friend warned me. "No one will respect you."
> Why would caring for a ward full of patients with multiple problems deserve less respect than caring for a ward full of the freshly angiogrammed? I once posed this question to a sub-specialist and he said, "There's less at stake." I asked what he meant. He said, "If you fuck up, it's not such a big deal...so I guess the thinking goes that a lesser physician can do the job."
> Half the patients in an acute care hospital are over the age of sixty-five... The single most important aspect of care is to have clinicians who *want* to look after this cohort...it doesn't matter who they are, as long as they have a desire to care for the elderly and feel there is a lot at stake. (Hitchcock 2015, pp.18–19)

The Australian Psychological Society has also noted this lack of status and perceived attractiveness about aged care as a career and suggests that this is a symptom of ageism in our society. In its 2000 position paper it says, "Research indicates that working in aged care is the least preferred option for trainee professionals such as medical and nursing students (Le Couteur, Bansal and Price 1997; Pursey and Luker 1995)"

(Australian Psychological Society 2000, p.4). It seems that whatever your profession, if you are working with older adults you could be viewed as not doing "serious" stuff. But, as the good doctor Hitchcock suggests, work related to elder care should be highly esteemed. It should not be viewed as "Mickey Mouse".

So, if you have not already, you might find yourself thinking that what you are doing is not "serious" psychotherapy. This reminds me of when a clinician who decided to enter our programme was shadowing me for a morning. He was a mental health social worker like me. I must admit, I did appreciate his honesty. Before we went in to see the first client of that day he said to me in hushed tones, "So, how much can you actually *do* with these people?"

We then went in to see a woman whom I had been meeting with for a while. She had a slight intellectual disability, was in her 70s, had multiple physical disabilities, and was mourning the loss of her husband. She and I settled into a familiar rhythm of working through her grief. It was slow work and I had the aid of a pack of picture cards. My "shadow" witnessed in this session the first set of tears that she had let herself shed for a very long time, and I saw him wipe his face a few times too.

After, he was speechless as we walked along the corridor. This veteran clinician appeared deeply moved. I wanted to encourage him to talk so asked how that was for him. We stopped and he said, "Yeah, that was full on," then he glanced at me and shook his head a little before adding, "that was *real* therapy," as if this was not what he had been expecting. I do not blame him for thinking like this. I get tempted to think like that myself sometimes – to think that what I am doing is a bit "Mickey Mouse".

But then I think of the delicate process of engagement, the topics of grief and trauma, communicating despite multiple disabilities, working in the facility context, dealing with family and others, having knowledge of the main dementias, adapting therapy to suit need, then modifying it even more so that it is in step with decline. Even work that I consider "informal" – and may *look* like just a pleasant chat – is every bit as intentional as the formal work that I do. Clinical psychologist Bob Knight, a leader in the field of psychotherapy with older adults, finds that when he is home visiting he needs to exude professionalism lest the transaction slip into the "too familiar" territory (Knight 2004). Perhaps that is why I do not take tea when in someone's private space.

But as well as presenting as a professional I think that it is important to believe just how much expertise you have. "What I am doing *rocks*!" Repeat this mantra to yourself; many times. You may not hear it from those around you.

Buttons and formal supervision
Transference and countertransference

Mr Fright is a softly spoken man in his late 70s. He only has good things to say about all his family. He is the sort of person that you cannot imagine even hurting a fly. In his younger days, you learn, he was an avid pool player and some awards adorn the ledge of his tiny room. You are seeing him because his wife, Janice, died suddenly two months ago. In sessions he alternates between emoting about his loss and appreciating the opportunity to drift into memories of yesteryear. Much of this relates to his love of pool and he has rattled off the games he enjoyed: eight-ball, three-ball, bank pool; and so it goes. But there is something you feel uneasy about. Something that seems to be coming in the way of your work with him; you just cannot put your finger on it. Then, one night, you have a dream and sit bolt upright in your bed. It was about your great-uncle Bob who was a scary alcoholic who loved playing pool. But, of course, you say to yourself: a classic case of countertransference. Freud would have had a field day!

The issue of transference and countertransference in work with older adults can have a negative effect on the therapeutic relationship if blind-spots are not acknowledged or dealt with (Knight 2004). The senior could channel irritations onto the therapist because they are in their 20s like others who have caused them grief. The client reminds the therapist of their mother or grandmother. The client finds it difficult to be guided by someone who reminds them of their son. The therapist finds it difficult to be advising someone who is their elder. All of these are "buttons" that can become more visible through peer or professional supervision and through a reflective practice which can address the problems created by these relational complexities.

Given that (in Australia at least) there are not many who work in a clinical capacity with advanced seniors it may be difficult to find mentors in this field related to your particular discipline. I have found that, while it is desirable to have professional guides familiar with this work, it is not essential. What is essential is that you respect the level of clinical competence from those whom you consult. They may have decades of experience as a counsellor or psychologist, they may have a similar therapeutic orientation to you, work in a related field such as palliative care, and be someone with whom you feel comfortable and can trust. You may have to educate them about the uniqueness of your work, the vulnerabilities that you could fall prey to, and what you would like them to look out for, but a trained supervisor or skilled clinician from any discipline or field should be adequate. Setting aside regular meetings (perhaps every eight weeks) with them is critical if you are to keep yourself fresh and your work effective.

The constancy of death and decline

Another "button" that you might find helpful taking to supervision is how you feel about death and decline. At the beginning of Chapter 6 it was suggested that our Western society can feel uncomfortable talking about death – or even thinking about it. While you can imagine that anyone going into aged care work would expect that their clientele is not going to get any younger or more able, the actual experience of death and decline can still be confronting at times. Remember that you are not just being with your client in an aged care facility, you are exposed to a whole array of sights and sounds. How does it feel to witness the lively man in the lounge room, over time, looking lost and without his spark? To be with someone who is mourning the loss of their lifetime lover? To have sessions with a delightful lady then, next time you visit, she is gone? Carer and nursing staff are exposed to this even more: one year sharing a hearty laugh with a cheeky soul and the next, trying to soothe their demented distress. They see the turntable of loss go round and around and around. While it is beyond the scope of this book to comment on the emotional needs of staff – which I believe is gathering in research interest – it does remind me of a story that I believe is also relevant for those who are geropsychologists and gerontological psychotherapists.

Her name was Lee. I met her at a social gathering and when she learnt that I was involved in aged care she explained how five years ago she graduated as a registered nurse. First she did hospital work. Then she found her way into aged care work. "I loved it!" she said, but there was something about how she paused to turn away that told me there was more to this story. She told me how respectfully caring for seniors fitted well with her family beliefs and culture and how she found the nursing work diverse and interesting – one minute attending to low blood pressure and the other navigating her way through a trillion medications. She liked the combination of a busy ward round with a homely feel. Each room she visited; expressions of a life story. Each resident a member of the facility's home. "But," she said to me, her glossy black hair slipping forward as her head slightly dipped, "it got too hard." "What did?" I asked. "People dying. It should not have got to me like it did."

Lee went on to explain to me how ashamed she felt of her grief when a resident died. How she loved the people entrusted in her care but how sad she was when death took them away or decline turned them into someone else. Was there anyone she spoke to about this, I wondered out loud. No, there was not. There was no onsite counsellor and she had not considered seeing an offsite one through the facility's Employee Assistance Programme. Lee spoke of an implied expectation that "the show must go on". Rooms were at a premium and a vacant one gets filled as quickly as a parking space in a busy city. We agreed on the practicalities of long-term care administration but I was struck by the depth of Lee's devotion and her sense of failure for feeling the way she did.

"Was not her sadness a sign that she cared?" I asked. She agreed that it was but, for perhaps a myriad of reasons, had also concluded that it had undermined her effectiveness. In the end, she decided to leave nursing for good. This 20-something woman, full of care and devotion, explained to me how she is trying to enjoy an administration position. "It does not give me people contact which I liked very much, but it does not make me upset either." Perhaps this change in career path was what Lee needed to do. But perhaps it was what she did not need to do had she had more support and was able to accept her humanity, use it even, instead of trying to beat it away.

Unfortunately, Lee is not alone in her shame and distress. It saddens me how many workers have confessed a silliness for feeling upset about a resident dying whom they were very fond of. "I shouldn't feel that way," they say hiding their face. In Chapter 6 you were introduced to the term "disenfranchised grief". This is exactly what is happening when staff feel ashamed to admit to feelings of loss for a resident. They reason that it is okay for family, okay for other residents but not okay for them as a paid worker. Is the same true for psychotherapists too? Well, as much as we might like to think we are more able than most to face this stuff, I suspect it is still relevant. Maybe more so. Maybe the less we think we are affected the more at risk we are of internally combusting like Lee and quitting for good? We need to always be honest (and kind) with ourselves. Is the experience of death and decline having an impact? Would it help to talk about it with someone – preferably a peer, a supervisor or external counsellor?

You might also like to ask yourself the following questions: Have you recently experienced a death in your family or friend circle? How many special people have died in your life? Are any of those a beloved grandparent who might be a little like an older adult you are working with? Have you personally cared for anyone who has been palliative? How does it feel to work with people facing similar issues? Do you find yourself feeling saddened by the prospect of ending up like the seniors who you consult – lonely, declining health, in a small room? And what about when their stories turn to the loss of loved ones – their children even? Do you find it hard to concentrate on your client when your heart has dashed off to those who you cherish? Do you tremble a little when you hear that word – death?

Managing your own distress

As with any other psychotherapeutic work, it can be helpful to acknowledge times when you are impacted personally. Being a counsellor or clinician with older people in care can be very emotional work. Part of what I love about psychotherapy is the intensity of it – you get to know someone very intimately – but it is impossible to be a sensitive person, like Lee was, and engage at this level without absorbing some emotion yourself. A reflective practice and professional supervision is essential, in my opinion, to ensure that you stay balanced between a healthy embracing of your humanness and a watchful eye on your own distress. The following are three strategies that I have personally found helpful in managing distress.

First, let yourself feel. By this I do not mean dissolving into tears in front of your client. They will soon start to doubt how well you can help them if you do! But do not bury your emotional reaction either. If what has been said has really touched you, especially if it has no links to your personal life, then letting a tear roll comfortably down your cheek can be a wonderful opportunity of validation. I have never forgotten what my placement supervisor once said when I was in my final year of social work, "It's okay to cry; just never more than your client." You can verbalize your own emotional reaction by saying something like, "This isn't small stuff is it? This is stuff that would have anyone feeling overwhelmed or upset," and you might find that this also will allow a generation not usually comfortable with emoting to get the release that they need. And be kind to yourself. Let yourself have a decent cry on your own or in supervision if what you have heard has been particularly heavy. Light a candle at home that night for a resident who has died – in honour of their life and your own feelings of appreciation and, maybe, distress. Jog just that bit harder during your exercise routine if there are feelings that need to be physically expressed. Share with your colleagues any pent-up emotion, quandary or existential question. We should not become robots. Our clients need us to stay human.

Second, if you have not developed a practice of meditation already, then I encourage you to try it as a way to deal with any dis-ease. In an instruction video for university students entitled *Introduction to Meditation*, Mark O'Donoghue, Buddhist practitioner and former psychotherapist, suggests that meditation is easier than most people think (UniThrive 2016). In this video Mr O'Donoghue goes on to explain that meditation is not about emptying your head of all your thoughts and working hard to relax. It is about choosing an object of focus (e.g. the breath in the nostrils) and developing your skills in attention by continually cycling through these four things: your object of focus, becoming distracted, noticing that you have become distracted, and gently returning your attention back to your object of focus.

Finally, a meditation practice – more specifically a mindfulness one – can help illuminate other issues that need addressing, perhaps in relation to countertransference. As alluded to earlier, when you are listening to the distressing circumstances of a senior it can have your heart dashing off to thoughts about people you love or your own circumstances. It can be easy just calling this "empathy" and justifying any strong emotional reaction to the pain that you are listening to as warranted. Well, yes – and no. Yes, using yourself as a reference point can illicit empathy and it would be impossible for our minds to be 100 per cent focused on the person in front of us all the time so some distraction is expected. But if strong emotions keep coming up for you with clients, then it might be because there are things in your own life that need to be dealt with. Your "empathy" might be less about you feeling your client's pain and more about feeling your own. A formal and/or informal mindfulness practice can get you in tune with your outer and inner experiences and help you take stock of your situation. By all means feel your client's pain but if the roads to your reflections keep leading back to *you* and not *them*, then this might be another good reason to trot off to supervision.

Compassion satisfaction

Have you ever been at a party and someone learns about what you do. "Oh god," they might say, "I don't know how you do it." It is as if, instead of learning that you are a counsellor, they have heard that you make ice blocks out of manure and then lick them. Well, personally, I do not know how teachers do the excellent work that they do, how my local checkout assistant can be so efficient, how facility staff stay chirpily engaged in endless routines of dressing and physical care. But I am eternally grateful that there are many out there who do! I want my children to receive quality education, I want to make my way through the checkout in a timely manner (and receive a pleasant smile) and I especially want to see aged care residents be attended to in the manner that they deserve. We all, as Jungian psychology suggests, have "gifts differing" (Briggs Myers and Myers 1995).

A few years ago I was reading the latest quarterly journal for my profession and I came across a wonderful phrase – compassion satisfaction. You have no doubt heard of compassion fatigue but this phrase flips things on its head. The article reported on qualitative research that looked into workers' experiences of trauma counselling and found out how therapists stay energized and thrive as they listen to multiple accounts of distress (Ling, Hunter and Maple 2014). They discuss how the literature refers to the negative *and* positive effects of indirect trauma experiences – that they can coexist – and relate this to other concepts such as "post-traumatic growth" and positive psychology (Figley 2002; Stamm 2002; Tedeschi and Calhoun 1995, 2004; all cited in Ling *et al.* 2014, p.298).

Four main themes resulted from their study. First they learnt how counsellors can find trauma work challenging and rewarding. This related both to interacting with complexity and an opportunity to provide valuable and meaningful work that fitted with a respondent's desire to help. Second, respondents spoke about using a number of strategies and drawing on personal characteristics or beliefs to help them navigate work that brought them in contact with adversity. They saw their emotional responses as reasonable and "By normalising and placing the responses in the context of empathy and compassion, participant counsellors were able to understand and therefore manage stress responses more effectively" (Ling *et al.* 2014, p.304). Third, participants made a conscious effort to limit their exposure to trauma work and engaged in reflective practices so that they could stay attentive to their needs and wellbeing. This last theme related to broader contexts such as receiving professional development. While "compassion satisfaction" was not *the* centre piece of the article, a number of worker strategies pointed toward this ability (Ling *et al.* 2014).

It seems that an important ingredient for staying fresh and engaged is in how you perceive your work. With advanced seniors it translates to zeroing in on how you are helping them and not on the extent of suffering. Instead of feeling exasperated by the degree of suffering, focus on what is in your control to try and alleviate it. I can feel far more satiated in a counselling session where I am actively facilitating release and change than I can sitting down to the nightly news which is full of images that I can do very little about. I am not saying that we must ignore signs of fatigue – recharging our batteries is essential – but could a session of mammoth despair also be one where you can see that your role is vitally appreciated? Is not that something to feel satisfied about? I see our work as "optimizers". No matter how big or bad, if we can make *the smallest* difference and improvement to someone's world then that is a cause of celebration. This attitude might also help to implicitly shift your client's view; look at what is needed to cope rather than on the suffering per se.

Dealing with frustrations and disillusions

Given how complex, and sometimes thankless, work with seniors can be it is no surprise that practitioners can feel a little blue or lose steam. While responding to challenge can be stimulating, the extent of challenge – individual and systemic – can become overwhelming. It is important to recognize this as a possibility and guard against it. We have already spoken about the importance of informal and formal supervision. That is one way to guard against frustrations and disillusions. The other is self-care and the following explores three ways to meet this need: recharging, diversity and disengagement.

What is the most effective thing for you to do to recharge your batteries? Do you prefer the company of others when feeling depleted or time to yourself? How able are you to "switch off" after the day has finished? What strategies help you do this the best? These are basic self-care issues but how often do we pause and reassess whether what we are doing is working for us or not? How often do we stop to look inwards and address tension and dis-ease? Learn to say "no". Work from home. Do regular exercise. Practise meditating – even just ten minutes a day. Get a massage. Let go of having a massive mortgage. Schedule time for yourself and those you care about. Keep yourself "well oiled" and do it without a sense of apology. This can be particularly difficult for women who have been strongly socialized into caring for others and who see acts of self-care as "selfish". If you were your own therapist, what might you say to your feelings of guilt? Might you ask if it is helpful or unhelpful? Might you explore ways to feel more free?

I have a confession to make. I would not like to be engaged in psychotherapy with older adults full time. I have found that diversity is an important strategy to offset issues of practice that can deplete my energy. For now, it is too difficult for me to ascertain how much this is the case for psychotherapy with older adults in Australia *at this particular point* in history or if I might feel this way with many conditions being different in time. What I do know is that my work with other age populations enables me to see therapy in a different light and it is just plain easier to deliver at times. I can more easily engage in mainstream modalities and apply new learning.

Overall, there is just less complexity to navigate and clients of younger generations are usually more motivated which brings with it an energy of its own. This is why I would caution against new counsellors starting off in aged care. I suspect it might be better to "cut your teeth" on more standard contexts of practice. With more experience you can then layer your skill set by adapting your training to work with seniors. But even so, mixing it up a bit is what works for me. Also, engaging in other pursuits such as training and (of course) writing.

Finally, I have known a number of veteran counsellors who have had to step out of work with older adults because it has just got too confronting, depleting or frustrating. I think it is far more wise to realize this than just keep struggling on. The work was not for them – at least not for now. This can be especially the case when caring for an elderly parent or family member yourself. Sometimes such disengagement is simply the need for a seasonal change. Once homeostasis has returned in some way, it can be a chance to re-engage. Whether it is a holiday or something a little longer, disengaging can bring with it a new perspective and new energy. And for those professionals who "hang in there", energy can also be found by surrounding yourself with others who are just as passionate about this work as you are and who know a little about the disempowering attitudes toward older adults that can infiltrate into the counselling context.

PERSONAL REFLECTION

1. Have you ever had a sense that working with an older adult population was somehow not "serious" psychotherapy?

_____

_____

2. What type of formal supervision do you currently engage in?

_____

_____

3. What "buttons" do you think you have/might have being a psychotherapist with advanced seniors?

_____

_____

4. How do you recharge? Do you struggle with guilt in looking after your own wellbeing?

_____

_____

5. Have you been or are you caring for a family member or friend?

_____

_____

CHAPTER 8

DISEMPOWERING ATTITUDES

I would like to remind you about our reference to Doctor Hitchcock in the preceding chapter, when considering the Mickey Mouse Mindset and work with seniors. Her reflections of working with seniors, and people engaged in that task, were that:

> The single most important aspect of care is to have clinicians who *want* to look after this cohort. Generalists, geriatricians, sub-specialists who've crossed to the dark side…it doesn't matter who they are, as long as they have a desire to care for the elderly and feel there is a lot at stake. (Hitchcock 2015, pp.18–19)

If you are reading this book it is highly likely that you are one such person who wants to care for seniors – and advanced seniors. The world needs more like you! Clearly, Doctor Hitchcock is another. Her essay "Dear life: on caring for the elderly" challenged our society's propensity to see old age as burdensome and irrelevant. She argued that ageism can still be seen almost everywhere you look – in our families, our social policies, in aged care facilities, in our health system and even in the very way that the older adults see themselves.

As a general physician in a large city public hospital in Australia she lifted the lid on the dismissive and downright disrespectful attitudes of her contemporaries that can have seniors be misunderstood and devalue their own life. She wryly pointed to a "too hard basket" attitude amongst her colleagues whenever a senior presents to a hospital: "…his or her arrival may set off a turf war. Doctors won't fight to take care of him; they'll fight not to" (Hitchcock 2015, p.15).

I must say, I do agree with this doctor's perception and experience. My own experience – at work and in life – has been that the way our Western society views ageing can be less than complimentary. As we reflected in Chapter 6 in the section "Readiness to die", our society, naturally, is geared toward an interest in life and can feel a little queasy when death stares us in the face. From the moment we are born we are moving toward progression, development, accumulation, productivity, and shoring up opportunities for health and wellbeing. When this progression cart starts rolling back the other way – toward obvious signs of ageing and decline – then our reflex response can be to try and slow it down. We do not like it. Every instinct in us tries to preserve, to progress. So it is little surprise that we do not take it kindly when forces of nature whittle the abilities of our bodies down.

If we, as a society, do not warmly embrace the concept of ageing or decline then it is not too much of a jump between this and having unhelpful (explicit or implicit) attitudes *toward* those who are ageing and declining. We might, justifiably, pride ourselves on our ability to have a non-judgemental approach to humans of all shapes and sizes, of all ages. But even the most saintly among us lives in a broader context and, in counselling, this translates to an awareness of the multitude of ways that ageist attitudes can be affecting your client – and even the counselling process itself or how you view your work.

In Chapter 7 we looked at how to guard ourselves, as psychotherapists working with advanced seniors, against disempowering mental frameworks – the Mickey Mouse Mindset – along with all manner of other frustrations and disillusionments. Staying interested and satisfied in work related to older adults is also about understanding the cultural milieu that surrounds you. What messages about older adults infiltrate the media, policies and general discussion? What social attitudes or beliefs might sap desire instead of fuel it? Being forewarned is to be forearmed. When we are able to see clearly through the mist of ageism we can be more alert to stories of prejudice or disempowerment and help our clients find a way to position themselves against such dominant discourses.

The following are five forms of ageism or attitudes that I suspect exist in our Western society:

- Ageist attitude #1: Urgh!

- Ageist attitude #2: "O" is for obsolete.

- Ageist attitude #3: It's not worth it.

- Ageist attitude #4: What do you expect?

- Ageist attitude #5: Where's the progression?

As this view is my humble opinion, not substantiated by research, I invite you to simply use my views to cross-reference with your own. These views are just the product of my experience; what about yours? Do they resonate? Do you disagree? Far from being a definitive set of beliefs – I am certain that there are positive beliefs in the community too – these propositions are to encourage reflection of your own observations rather than to persuade your opinion. But whatever your conclusions may be, you might agree with me on the following point: attitudes on ageism should embrace the opposite. Respectful approaches to ageing would then include:

- #1: Not finding old age distasteful.

- #2: Not "writing people off" just because they are old.

- #3: Believing that seniors are worth it.

- #4: Trying to treat what is treatable.

- #5: Valuing quality of life over a person's ability to progress or be "productive".

If I have assumed wrongly of you then I do apologize. You are welcome to take your own personal orientation on all that I present. To aid this presentation, and reflect on the opposite of what might be an ageist stance, we will refer back to Harold in "ageist attitude #2" whose story you have been following throughout this book. You are invited to continue imagining how your work with Harold, and his wife Elizabeth, is unfolding. You will also be encouraged to imagine how your work as a psychotherapist with them is embodying a respectful practice in how it is alert to, and actively positioning against, ageist attitudes that might be evident in the surrounding social fabric.

Ageist attitude #1: Urgh!

I loved opening up the *Weekend Australian* magazine one lazy Saturday morning to find local Byron Bay identity "Feather" staring back at me in a skimpy bikini proudly displaying nearly every bit of her weather- and life-worn 78-year-old body. She was photographed by

Natalie Grono for the 2015 National Photographic Portrait Prize and made her way as a finalist. Feather (and Natalie) did not end up winning the Portrait Prize but she won my heart.

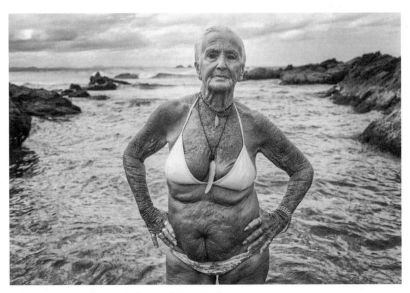

Figure 8.1: Feather and the Goddess Pool
Reproduced by permission of the photographer

I am sure I was not alone in my appreciation of the way Feather stared self-assuredly down the camera lens but my family brought me back to the real world. "Urgh!" my 14-year-old son exclaimed as he spied the picture, "That's ugly!" and he pleaded for me to spare him the image that was spoiling his breakfast. Had Feather been a 20-something Ferrari model I am sure his response would have been somewhat different. So, what teenage boy would want to see an old lady in a bikini, I hear you say. True. But is his reaction representative of a general distaste for "old"?

If we did not have an aversion to "old" then how many more advertisements would there be where seniors, instead of fresh-faced young things, are used to promote a product? You might see a senior selling a pre-paid funeral, perhaps, or a retirement unit, but how sexy is it? How much do we relish the maturity of age versus the fountain of youth? How longingly do we look at the truth of an ageing body? In Buddhism an old person is believed to be a heavenly messenger. Why? Because, as the teaching goes, one is reminded of how unhelpful it can be to feel shocked, humiliated or disgusted at such a sight for this will one day be their destiny (Fella 2009). To deny the inevitability of age is to stay locked in a state of suffering; trying to hold onto a Peter Pan life of "forever young" when reality speaks of something else. Perhaps the "Urgh!" is less about the older person per se that we see and more what they represent, the confronting truth of our own destiny?

Feelings of repulsion may also fuel negative stereotypes about seniors. What might start as a reaction to something "old" becomes a blinkered appraisal for all in that category. Advanced seniors can be lumped into one large melting pot of "Urgh!" without an interest to offset negative attitudes with positive ones. One study that examined the judgements people make about older adults discovered that negative stereotypes were more commonly associated with those over 80 than for those in the younger senior age group (Hummert *et al.* 1995).

Attempts to offset unhelpful stereotyping can be seen in the creation of the contextual, cohort-based, maturity, specific-challenge model (CCMSC) that you were introduced to in Chapter 2. It aims to view adult development in more positive terms than the more traditional loss-deficit model of ageing (Knight 2004). It encourages a closer look, an appreciation of many nuances, that can make up the experience of an older adult. And the tenets of positive psychology further fuel an interest in turning around feelings of despair or disgust so that panoramas of hope and appeal come into view. The process of ageing can then be seen as fruitful: of gaining wisdom, of being clear about one's identity, of thriving despite physical decline, of making the most out of any situation, of taking life firmly by both hands and never letting go until your time is up.

Counselling can also be an avenue to turn the "Urgh!" inclination around. First, as a gerontological psychotherapist you can be on guard against any attitudes that may undermine what you do – the Mickey Mouse Mindset – and actively appreciate the significance of working with a senior cohort. Second, you can be on the lookout for how your clients might become entrapped with disempowering attitudes about their age and stage in life. Could it be that societal judgements are enlarging feelings of despair or self-disgust when this need not be so?

Third, you can actively challenge any internal recoil at the idea of exploring the intimate – the sexual. Ph.D. candidate Alison Rahn from the University of New England has co-authored the paper "Conflicting agendas: the politics of sex in aged care" and found in her research that addressing the sexual needs of aged care facility residents is often shunned (in Smith 2016). Specifically she notes that "…it is often the staff who prevent couples from intimacy. The culture in aged care facilities also exists because most of the staff tend to be young and of course the residents are old and it is inconceivable, revolting or impossible to think that couples would want intimacy" (in Smith 2016, p.1). True, members of "the lucky generation" may not be leaping into a conversation of this type but how much space are we creating for this in our transactions? Perhaps an initial "Urgh!" can become a more neutral and curious "Oh?" And finally, you can pay extra attention to seeing your clients as individuals instead of succumbing to polarizations of "dotty and difficult" or "sweet and lovely". These groupings can blinker workers to important nuances of positivity or discourage clients to step outside of limiting identities.

Ageist attitude #2: "O" is for obsolete

Harold considers you for a minute before replying, "I'm falling to bits. Look at me." It is a candid comment. Not laced with the despair of months gone by but, you note, not filled with hope either. Could it be more related to grief or a feeling of uselessness? You are not sure so you take your opportunity and explore some more. "What do you mean by that?" you ask. He does not work properly anymore, you learn; what good is he to anyone? Oh, yes, he quickly adds, Elizabeth loves him and he her, but just generally? His voice floats off.

The familiar hum of facility life infiltrates the room as you continue your exploration on how he feels about this ageing business. He has not mentioned his feelings about this before. So focused have sessions been on more immediate issues: getting more sunlight in, getting out of bed, dealing with past demons, managing the more intrusive ones of the present, identifying key values, celebrating a long life and nurturing his relationship with his wife Elizabeth. Much has been achieved and he is certainly more engaged in his world than when you first saw him. But today – at session 12 – there are stones yet unturned.

You and he consider how, maybe, his views are influenced by the messages in the wider community. Is there a difference in how we view youth versus age, you wonder out loud. Yes, perhaps there is, he replies but the philosophical plane does not seem to be his preference. You remember his love of cars. How should vintage cars be treated, you venture. "With respect!" he shoots back. You happily agree on this point and ask if he thinks older adults who may no longer work so well are treated like vintage cars or feel as though they belong on the scrap heap. This hits home. "The scrap heap," he says. While the analogy is not perfect it allows for connection and insight. You spend the rest of the session talking about how he loved to restore old cars and how "old" does not have to mean "obsolete". How else could we think about age, you enquire. What aspects of maturity can he appreciate in himself? How can he still feel a valued member of our society even if his body does not work so well anymore?

A close cousin of "Urgh!" is the attitude we have about things that are old and worn out. We live in a throw-away society. You only have to meander through the streets when hard rubbish is being collected to see evidence of this: chairs, tables, kids' toys, bikes, plant pots, many of which are not technically broken but that are old and no longer wanted. And the reality is that planned obsolescence is now a cornerstone of our economic society. Much as we might not want to replace and dispose, many of us have little choice. Your eight-year-old washing machine stops working. What to do? Shell out a lot of money to try and fix it or spend not much more on a brand new one?

Bernard London (1932) first came up with the term "planned obsolescence" in his pamphlet *Ending the Depression through Planned Obsolescence*. Ever since then, and after gaining gusto in the 1950s, manufacturers have embraced the trend to have a built-in shelf life for their product to ensure turnover in production. Couple this with a consumerist society where "yesterday's fashion" is a euphemism for "seriously backward" and you get a culture that celebrates the new and the shiny.

In the information technology world, replacement has become less of a fashion choice and more a necessity. You *have* to get the upgrade if you still want to run a business, have a job or continue to do what you need to. Of course interest in our environment now challenges manufacturers and consumers alike to be more eco-friendly; we now try and "think green" where our resources – economic or otherwise – allow. Children's movies such as *Robots* and *WALL-E* encourage the next generation to be less materialistic and more sustainable in their choices but upgrades and replacements when things get old are the life that we live now.

Even if we have the best of intentions, "old" can become synonymous with "obsolete". What does this mean for how we view other things when they are old? People when they are old? Was this what Harold was struggling with in the above example? Of course, the goodwill in us might rile against any such notion that our consumerist habits could generalize out to how we view something precious – a living thing – but is there an element of this attitude that seeps through our consciousness?

As much as we might want to hold onto life is there also a part of our society that looks disdainfully on "goods that are past their use-by date". The words of Doctor Hitchcock come to mind again: "My chief aim is to strike a note of caution and to make explicit something that often remains unsaid and yet can be heard quite clearly: that the elderly are burdensome, bankrupting, non-productive. That old age is not worth living" (Hitchcock 2015, p.4).

If we are to work with seniors we need to actively examine our attitudes to "old" and how they have a tendency to become synonymous with "obsolete". This does not mean that you have to love everything old and tut-tut all that is new. I am certainly no lover of antique shops or 1980s sound tracks (you might be). What is important is to be cognizant of how society's values can affect our own, and can come unbidden into our therapeutic encounters or be present in how our clients view themselves.

Ageist attitude #3: It's not worth it

Jessie J, British singer and songwriter, tells us, "It's not about the money, money, money", and to forget about the price tag. Well, true, it would be good if it was not about the money. But the back story of what our culture values can be very much about the money when it comes to how we view seniors and how important their psychological health is to us. Allow me to be quite frank with you: what is the return on investment?

In the business world you need to make money if you want to survive. New ventures get backed by investors if they can put a good business case up which suggests a good return on investment. It does not matter if you are selling safety gloves or wanting to open up a new restaurant – if you have done your market research and you have a good chance of success then your idea is likely to be seen as worth it. Moreover, businesses with a proven track record of making a profit and satisfying customer need will be applauded as successful. If they make it into *Fortune* magazine their product and business model will be seen as even more valuable.

It is the same in the human services and in the medical community. Services, research or organizations that are seen as making a positive contribution to society are often those seen as worth it. Programmes that make a difference or are valued in the community are the ones more likely to attract the funds needed in order to ensure their survival. But what we, as a society, deem as worth our investment is complex and interesting. Which vulnerable populations do we sympathize with the most? Maybe some causes that we invest in are topical – a bushfire or hurricane appeal. Maybe some causes attract our sympathies for personal reasons – we lost our sister to breast cancer or an uncle to a brain tumour. How do we feel about children who are suffering?

As a social worker, psychotherapist, mother and human being I applaud all efforts in benefiting the wellbeing of humanity. I am not asking you to justify where your allegiances lie but I would like to point out how some populations may not reach the radar of our sympathies as easily as others. I suggest to you that we are at our most sympathetic when people are cut down in their prime or not even allowed to reach an age where they could realize any potential. And what about when there *is* potential, like job support programmes or counselling for populations who have scope to be productive citizens and eventually earn their own way?

Where do seniors fit in here, especially advanced seniors? Well, that is a very good question. They are at the end of the road of their productivity. They have had their prime and realized, as best they could, their potential. Do they, even themselves, feel like they are worth any attention other than to the basics? What about Harold? Do you think that he has been struggling with a sense of worth – of value?

In my experience a proportion of the current cohort of older adults do not feel like they are worth the trouble. Why is that? I suspect that it has something to do with the way we construct "value". Our society places a lot of emphasis on productivity as it links to financial gain. Unpaid labour is not as valuable as paid labour. If you doubt this then I invite you to speak to any new mother who has gone from successful career girl to full-time bum-wiping stay-at-home mum. As a psychotherapist who also specializes in issues related to maternal health I can tell you that women now often do not feel as valued in their role as mother as they do in a role that pays. The more lucrative the job, the more a sense of prestige is realized – and mourned when it is not there. "Mummy wars" flourish between the paid workers and the stay-at-homes, and central to these unhelpful feuds is the concept of value or worth.

Seniors today, especially ones in aged care facilities, often confess to me that they do not feel productive anymore, valued. They say this as if someone might fine them for uttering such nonsense but the gravity in their tone is unmistakable. They are shut away, lonely and no longer feel as though they are valuable contributing members of society. Perhaps as well as the "stolen generations"[22] we have, with a number of older adults, the "forgotten generation" too.

Of course aged care facilities try and offer a sense of productivity through lifestyle activities but the fact remains, their sense of productivity has been neutered. Perhaps if they we were still a part of a tribal or farming community their wisdom and presence might be more valued, and visible, but there is little scope in our society for seniors to feel included and worth it. Even the idea of counselling them can challenge our commercial sensitivities: how would our society benefit? Is it worth it?

Ageist attitude #4: What do you expect?

We can be tough on each other when a softer attitude might be more kind. "What do you expect?!" we might say (laughing of course) to a new parent who is not getting much sleep. We seem to say this more during life's transitions than for anything else – baby blues, teenager troubles, marital weariness after 30 years – and we say it (or at least think it) for ageing too. Got trouble walking and you are 80? "Get over it, gramps. You're old!"

But what is often overlooked in these so-called humorous quips to hardship is that beneath the jocular interchange can lie deep rivers of loss and disenfranchised grief. What does it mean to no longer feel human due to sleep deprivation; to live in a constant war zone of argument with your teenager; to not be excited by your beloved anymore? What does it mean to not be able to walk to the shops because of your dicky knee? To no longer be independent? To rely on others where once you were strong and able?

When we age we can expect that things do not work so well anymore but that does not mean that we like it. The "What do you expect?" attitude can have a silencing effect on experiences of loss related to transition or natural decline. It can also come in the way of attempts to rectify dysfunction that is perfectly likely to respond to treatment – whether it be a dicky knee or depression.

"Well," Harold had said in response to his Geriatric Depression Scale score, despondently but still with a hint of incredulity, "What do you expect?" Yes, you think to yourself, one would expect to feel miffed at having the rug of life completely ripped out from underneath you but – "When people have gone through something like you," you had said to him, "then, yes, you can expect a fair amount of grief and even depression. But equally it can be easy to think that just because you are over 80 and things aren't the same anymore that depression is just something one has to put up with. The good news is, you don't need to." For this regular bloke – your client – your words were like him sampling a smoked salmon canape: not really repulsive but not that familiar either.

When the tentacles of ageism touch even the aged themselves, a state the APS call "internalised ageism" (APS 2000, p.5), and are coupled with a dose of "grin and bear it" style fortitude, then people like Harold can have a hard time warming to the idea that life need not be quite so tough. You might need to frequently massage your conversations with realistic hope and self-compassion to give your client another avenue to consider. "Depression is not a normal part of ageing," you might say. Or "Everyone has the right to quality of life no matter how old you are." But it can take a while before this sense of permission filters through.

I once saw a woman in her 90s who lived in her own home and was trying to find her place in the world after her husband had died. She also had a sore knee and, while she still had a car and licence, could no longer drive due to the pain. A scooter enabled her to take care of the basics but getting around in her car gave her social connection and independence – that she was sorely missing. "Had you considered an operation?" I asked. She had, but had her reservations. "I don't want to make a fuss," she countered. But the discomfort of her knee kept her awake at night and cast a shadow on how long she might be able to live at home. Aged care facility living was definitely not on her agenda but her knee was starting to force her hand.

Then, I learnt that she finally saw the specialist to discuss a knee replacement. "I wouldn't advise that," he had apparently said. "Why?" she had asked. "Well, it's your age. There could be complications and, well, you're 91." Buoyed by our discussion on her right to pursue quality of life issues no matter the age, she persisted and went ahead with surgery. After the operation, and having made a full recovery, she was elated. "I can do so many more things now that I got my knee fixed up!"

Of course sometimes protesting about decline or dysfunction brings about more suffering than the actual object of contention but if improvement is possible then it should be entertained. Our society can have expectations about ageing that reinforce a "grin and bear it" attitude when a more prudent or kind one might be to look at what one need not have to put up with. Guarding against the "What do you expect?" attitude means entertaining hope and encouraging intervention for experiences that are treatable and are having a negative effect on quality of life.

Ageist attitude #5: Where's the progression?

As you turn your car into the facility parking lot you stop for a moment after the engine cuts. You think of the three residents you need to see at this home but one has made a particularly indelible mark. Harold. It was not that he took to therapy like a duck to water, but it was his plain spirited perseverance despite it not being his "happy place" that endeared you to him all the more. How brave he has been to step into the world of psychotherapy – of baring his soul like men of his era tend not to. And Elizabeth. She has been as much of a helper as one whom you have gladly helped.

Both have progressed, as a couple, and as individuals. You admire how Harold has knuckled down to getting from life what he can. From finding pleasure despite his circumstances – like the sight of a flower thrusting itself through the cracked desert floor. Where once low mood had thrown him into a prison cell and slammed the door shut, now he has found the key to his freedom and is learning to find meaning in the land of change that he was unceremoniously dumped onto.

Harold is getting better and therapy will soon conclude, you think to yourself as you sign yourself in at reception. This idea will not surprise him today. You have prepared him for it – spoken of the progress noted. Today you intend to assess him again. Your programme requires pre/post assessments. "It's just part of the new funding requirements," your manager had explained, "all the other programmes are required to record this data too." At least you are allowed to use a "senior-friendly" instrument. At session two you had used the Emotion Thermometers and the high score, mostly eights out of ten, had prompted you to administer the GDS. Harold certainly seems a completely different person to when you first met with him so a score that indicates progress today is highly likely.

As you gently tap on Harold's door and enter you are surprised to see Elizabeth there. She knows that this is your appointment time and you have already spent time with them as a couple and her individually. Is something the matter? But your brain has barely registered this question before the answer is clear. Yes. Harold is back to being in bed and his eyes look watery. You sit silently down and listen as, mainly Elizabeth, explains how Ralph – Harold's best mate – died suddenly of a heart attack two days ago. Oh. This is very sad news and poor Harold is really upset. Clearly, no assessment measures will be completed today. It is not the fact that a high score is likely again due to this change in circumstance; it is that Harold's need of support right now trumps any paperwork – and ideas of closure – you might have planned.

For people like Harold, the experience of loss can hit like a tsunami. While someone who is palliative knows about wave after wave of loss and decline – older adults can be exposed to this for reasons that extend beyond their own circumstance. Not only may they have had to say goodbye to a beloved pet, be living somewhere that they would rather not, feel as if their identity and independence have been cut down, but by virtue of them being an advanced senior (no matter how their body is fairing) they can be exposed to loss on a grand scale. People around them are old too. They might not only be noticing loss and decline in others, seeing favourite carers leave, saying goodbye to mates they have befriended in long-term care, but also have people very dear to them die. A husband or wife. A best friend of over 70 years.

How would that be for you, do you think? Might it be a little like a child having just built a fantastic LEGO® creation only to have his brother come along and knock parts of it over? You see, whatever amazing work you might have done to help your client cope with one situation, you cannot prevent the waves of many other losses come crashing to their shore. Sure, other populations ebb and flow with the life challenges set before them, but rarely are they straddling parallel roads that are travelling toward their decline *and* change or losses that relate to events external to them. How is progression to be found here? Glowing signs that your programme is effective? And how might evaluation measures feel to someone whose life is coloured with such loss? Could indications that distress is still high feel like an inadequacy in them (at best an inadequacy of therapy) when really it just is what it is? Life at the "bugger" end of things? Why is the clinical world so fascinated with assessment beyond using it to aid case conceptualization?

Perhaps it has something to do with the agenda behind psychotherapy. If you are not working toward some type of improvement then what is the point? It may be short-term solution-focused intervention or it may be longer-term psychotherapeutic work. But the overarching goal is to move toward a situation where the client feels better about their situation, more empowered to meet life's challenges, with less symptomology.

Perhaps it also links to the importance of quantifying progression in the evidence-based world of psychological theory. The logic goes something like this: the more a theory or intervention can show significant progress based on a set of measures designed by those researching it, then the more credible that intervention is in medical, academic and clinical circles. The more credible a theory is, the more likely it is to be approved by the health care system of your locality (i.e. Medicaid, the National Health Service or Medicare) and seen as the gold standard for use by practitioners. Likewise, programmes that can substantiate progression or effectiveness have a better chance of continued funding if they can prove their worth. It all makes good sense.

Good sense for work with other populations, maybe, but not good sense for advanced seniors. For other populations this model of service delivery justified through progression may also be less relevant. Those who are palliative might not have fabulous post scores on a quantitative measure but, through qualitative means, their appreciation of therapy or greater sense of ease could shine through. In these instances, therapeutic engagement accommodates for decline, and evaluation of effectiveness is not so focused on progression as such but of finding meaning and experiencing support. Similarly, therapy for those with chronic mental health issues is encouraged to manage episodes of heightened instability rather than aiming for significant progression. But even for these two groups, as outlined before, the internal and external circumstances are often still not as challenging as end of life for an older adult.

While I would like to stress that progression – noticeable signs of sustained improved mood – certainly can be noted amongst an older adult clientele, and not all feel knocked down by their circumstances, for the most part counselling advanced seniors sits in a context of (often significant) decline. Any gains that you make may be blown away by another tornado of loss: their wife just died, their animal had to be put down because there was no one to care for it, they had another fall, their favourite carer moved interstate. In the case of Harold it was that his best mate just died. The list can be endless and, for people at this stage in life, a number of losses can happen all at once.

Counsellors who are too focused on progression can feel disheartened and give up easily. The work is similar to palliative care or living with a serious illness in that expectations of "outcomes" need to be balanced against what is realistic considering the enormity of what someone is experiencing. Certainly, just being a listening ear and helping people reframe the way they view their circumstances can counter a snowballing decline in psychological health but in the words of Amaranth Foundation's CEO, mental health social worker and life-limiting illness expert Julianne Whyte OAM, intervention is more about "care not cure" (personal communication 2013).

It is understandable to be interested in progression, we can base our satisfaction and worth as a counsellor on such things, but there is much at stake if we subscribe to glossy expectations of improvement too much. Not only can our morale and interest take a nose dive but we may also unwittingly project a sense of hopelessness or failure (ours or theirs) onto the client. We might despair at measures at the end of therapy that look worse than at the beginning. We might unconsciously imply that the client is not being positive enough or side with them in their self-recriminations that if only they could look on the bright side more. How would that attitude help their situation?

What can be more helpful and respectful is taking a look at this notion of progression and re-badging it. What if we looked at our work in terms of optimization instead of progression? What if instead of trying to find pre/post quantitative measures we took a shorter-range focus or more qualitative feedback on how therapy is beneficial? It might be a moment when their eyes soften and they say with relief, "thank you". It might be the tears welling up that tell you your reflections are spot on. It could be a response to what that session meant to them and you might hear things like "I felt listened to for the first time in my life" or "I don't feel so silly anymore" or "It's the only time when I don't feel like I have to pretend."

They are outcomes in my opinion yet, overall, they may not stand out after another wave of loss has crashed to the shore. If we see progression more as moments of optimization – that may or may not be captured on a psychological measure or feedback form – then we may find that there are more veins of gold in the rock of their decline than we had first supposed. Veins of gold that can be good for both worker and client to mine and appreciate for how it sparkles.

PERSONAL REFLECTION

1. What ageist attitude/s have you noticed the most in society?

_____

_____

2. Which attitude are you most aware of in your contact with older adults?

_____

_____

3. Which one do you think is most likely to be "invisible" to you and why?

_____

_____

4. How might you protect yourself and therapy from unwittingly being complicit toward an ageist attitude?

_____

_____

5. What do you most like about the idea of working with advanced seniors?

_____

_____

CHAPTER 9

BUILDING SENIOR-FRIENDLY CARE SYSTEMS

Building senior-friendly care systems and being senior friendly is more than just wanting to work with older adults. It is about taking an honest look, inside and out, at what might sabotage a truly respectful practice. Practising holism. What personal and systemic barriers get in the way of creating therapeutic spaces that allow seniors to thrive? And not thrive according to a set of values that we, of the younger generation, have ordained as "healthy", but according to the values that seniors themselves see as worthy? How can we balance our duty of care sensibilities with client need? How can we provide relevant programmes of specialist care that are not at the mercy of a "one size fits all" approach to funding and practice? How can we create attractive opportunities to maximize worker interest and cultivate service delivery options that are accessible on many levels? How can psychotherapeutic intervention contribute to a reclaiming of senior status and an interest in consulting them? How can we bring "sexy back" to the practice of acknowledging our elders for the wisdom they hold within?

Tanner and Harris (2008) in their work with older adults also believe in the importance of taking a holistic approach. In doing so, they refer to how Lloyd (2002) defines holism:

> Holism is not concerned solely with the whole person, it is concerned with whole systems and *wholeness*, in both persons and systems and the interactions between them... A holistic approach to the assessment and meeting of the needs of individuals requires focus on the social structures which shape their lives and the mechanisms which impact upon their experiences of services. (Lloyd 2002, p.166, in Tanner and Harris 2008, p.144)

Therefore, being senior friendly in work with older people is about going beyond the individual and examining wholeness in and between multiple system levels, which is what this chapter hopes to explore.

Empowerment or dependency?

It is a legitimate request. You are asked to see Mrs Wish because she has become more withdrawn of late. You take a shine to Mrs Wish, a former school teacher, and her astute observations of her predicament. According to Mrs Wish, her withdrawal from other residents is a pragmatic option to preserve her sanity. "How many times can I make felt decorations with a bunch of people who don't even know where they are?!" You see her point. "You see," Mrs Wish explains, "I'm fine here" – she points to her head – "just not here" – her hand waves over the rest of her body. She talks about not wanting to be a burden for her family – that is why she chose to live in this facility – and also how all her friends have now died. "It's just me," she says looking straight at you.

When she lived at home she used to be a member of a book club and relished the weekly analysis and social contact. Transport issues, physical decline and eyesight problems put an end to this pursuit. Hearing loss also makes phone contact difficult. Face to face seems to work well though, you note. In sum, she is lonely and intellectually deprived. Her eyes light up when you walk in the room. "Oh good!" she often exclaims. "Finally someone interesting to talk to!" She tells you that she loves how you help her think about things, reflect back and cause her to reappraise. Staying focused on any one goal is a problem though. As much as you try and work toward change she keeps cleverly diverting your attention with a new issue, laments that she has lost the note from last session, or apologizes for not letting you follow your agenda. Is that what I'm doing, you ask yourself, following my agenda and not hers? And so, you are invited into conversations that seem less interested in solving anything than simply having conversation.

> On the one hand this work is easy. All you have to do is be a sounding board. On the other hand it is very challenging: How are therapeutic goals being upheld here? How much am I creating dependency by continuing to offer a compassionate ear? How can I conclude therapy and Mrs Wish not feel abandoned or rejected? On what grounds could I conclude it if it appears to be so beneficial? How long can this go on for? Am I neglecting other clients that need therapy too? Am I misappropriating the use of money that funds this programme?

The vast majority of seniors that I see are incredibly lonely and starved of opportunities for meaningful conversation. The therapeutic context can be seen as a wonderful saviour for their predicament: it can provide regular in-depth contact with another human being and can be deeply satisfying on an intellectual and emotional level. It can relieve boredom in spectacular ways. Whether they are playing by "the rules of therapy" or not may be of little consequence to them. Through fair means or foul they can orchestrate engagement in ways that deliciously ignite their soul and mind (and self-esteem). What does it mean to be "senior friendly" when you suspect that therapy is more a means for social or intellectual engagement than any interest to work toward change? This is a thorny question and one that I do not profess to hold a definitive answer to but, I believe, response pathways do deserve to be entertained.

Addressing dependency – on therapy or any health service – is not a new concept and certainly not limited to the population of older adults. But with older adults there are unique issues that can cloud a therapist's judgement. First, continuation of therapy could inadvertently be meeting more the therapist's need than the client's. Second, disempowering constructs can have both parties not questioning roles that perpetuate a paternalistic and "needy" involvement. Third, the therapeutic context may be the only deeply satisfying human encounter that the older person is connected to.

Therapist need

Knight (2004) points to the very common dilemma for therapists to find it difficult concluding therapy with an older client. Perhaps an element of countertransference is evident in the above example. Maybe Mrs Wish is not as lonely as you think and will not miss therapy nearly as much as you think she might. Maybe the problem lies more in your discomfort about ending therapy than hers: your overinflated view about how beneficial therapy is to that pers on and a sense of overwhelm about all the difficulties they are facing. Maybe Mrs Wish will cope just fine if you signal for closure – despite her appreciation of your visits. We can forget to leave room for the client's own ability in solving their problems. Seniors, especially, have a very long life to draw on in terms of coping with life's adversities. They may not like many elements of life now but their assessment of reality may not be as bleak as yours. Hence, by just letting therapy roll on with no end in sight could prevent someone like Mrs Wish discovering her own resources and putting into practice what therapy has illuminated to her.

Perpetuating a "needy" context

At the opposite end of the ageism spectrum is "anti-ageist positivism" (Bytheway 1995, p.128) which generates sickly sweet views about older adults and can lead to dependency. Co-dependency between an older adult and their caretaker/s can unwittingly exploit vulnerabilities in the senior and feed an appetite of insecurity in the person providing care. Given that therapeutic contexts often intimately explore a client's situation and require deep trust for this to flourish, care needs to be taken that therapy does not just become a substitute for co-dependency where both client and therapist bask in the glow of a paternalistic and disempowering relationship. Being senior friendly in this context means regular supervision to ensure that you are not meeting any subversive need of your own to be a "knight in shining armour" to those in your care. You could ask yourself how you feel about your client appreciating you versus therapy and see if a level of warmth arises for the former. If so, then it might be time to redirect focus back to what *therapy* can provide so you can better see when therapy has completed its course and it is time for you to leave.

Insatiable need

Maybe you have guessed right: Mrs Wish is not into therapy as much as she is with having a decent conversation with someone who can remember their name. While there are often restrictions on how many sessions a client may receive – under the Australian national health care system the limit each calendar year is ten – this may not stop your client from repeatedly getting their medical practitioner to refer to you because they like your company. And if you are a part of a programme that leaves session number to the discretion of the worker, the downside to this largely advantageous scenario is knowing when the therapeutic relationship is no longer a means to an end but an end in itself. Need of it is insatiable and likely only to strengthen over time. In this instance conversations that explicitly acknowledge the benefit – and potential loss – of the therapeutic relationship can be helpful. Sensitivity is needed in tabling the often very real fact that therapy is their sole source of meaningful connection and the absence of it yet another grief to endure.

Trying to prevent such a situation is difficult. It can be impossible to detect early on and discussion about the parameters of therapy may not be absorbed or remembered. I find it best to manage on a case by case basis: be honest about your concerns, give plenty of warning about closure and work toward it systematically (maybe also counting down the agreed session number), pre-empt future challenges and explore loss sensitively, create some ceremony on the last session (a card, a therapeutic letter) and maybe schedule a follow-up visit a few months down the track but be clear about the intention that contact is not to be ongoing. Having said this (and done these things) I still find the decision of how long to let a client utilize therapy a difficult one when they clearly get benefit from the relationship. Being senior friendly can mean appreciating the often very fine line between empowerment and dependency when therapy is the only available choice for deep social fulfilment.

Relevant programmes of specialist care

Oscar Wilde (1894) once said, "The old believe everything, the middle-aged suspect everything, the young know everything." While many factors can affect one's outlook or perception – age is one of them. And age can also affect the different needs we might have. When you are 20 you are not likely to be scouring the supermarket shelves for the best value in continence pads but when you are 70 you might be! A product relevant for one age bracket might not be so relevant for another. The same is true for a service or a model that underpins that service. Being senior friendly in response to life change and distress for older adults means that all elements of service delivery should be examined for their ability to be relevant: the initial engagement approach, the intervention and relationship, internal programme contexts and external socio-political contexts. Figure 9.1 highlights this matrix and the following expands on each element.

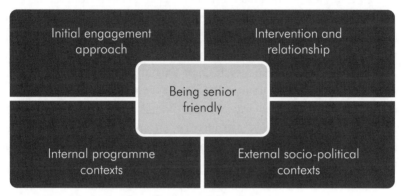

Figure 9.1: The senior-friendly service delivery matrix

Initial engagement approach

If the aim of psychology is to "…be attentive to the consequences of ageism, stereotyping and pathologising of older persons' experiences, and to adopt wherever possible principles of empowerment, respect, and recognition of the diversity and complexity of those experiences" (APS 2000, p.3) then it makes sense to scrutinize the way in which seniors are engaged when they first come in contact with a psychological service. Is language being used that they understand and feel comfortable with? In Chapter 2, you were introduced to the generational nuances that our current cohort of advanced seniors seem to possess which included an unfamiliarity with counselling contexts – even the word "wellbeing". Later language was, again, referred to as either engaging or alienating; empowering or disempowering. For example, describing your sessions as a "chat" was considered more relevant to this cohort than "therapy", words like "change" more appropriate than "psychological symptoms". And you were encouraged to move away from a focus on pathology or stigma by not using words or phrases such as "geriatric", "behavioural deficits", "failed to progress" or "disorder".

In Chapter 4 the over-use of formal assessment was questioned and in Chapter 5 informal and implicit contexts of biographical enquiry were suggested as a more preferred entry point than explicit forms of engagement common in typical therapeutic exchanges. Described as an "undercover agent" this chapter proposed five guiding principles for any psychological contact with a senior, especially when they are hearing of your service for the first time: dignity, choice, value, trust and a permission to talk. Reminiscence Therapy style approaches can create better understanding, contribute to trust and generate self-worth (Tanner and Harris 2008, p.141). These person-centred biographical conversations can be essential starter points *before* visits or sessions adopt a more traditional psychology flavour – especially when the senior is not grasping your collar asking you to fix their emotional distress but is experiencing distress nonetheless. But a life story investigation or interview can also be, in and of itself, therapeutic for the way it takes on strong flavours of Narrative Therapy. Through the process of re-engaging a senior in their life history and elevating them as expert in these knowledges, opportunities can be created that subjugate unhelpful self-definitions and allow for rich descriptions of alternative stories.

Intervention and relationship

An impressive body of research is developing with regard to the evaluation of psychotherapeutic practices for older adults and Cognitive Behavioural Therapy stands out as a consistent high performer, especially in the management of depression (Secker, Kazantzis and Pachana 2004; Wells *et al.* 2014). Psychologists, in particular, are interested in such scientific evaluations and only in implementing evidence-based practices that demonstrate strong efficacy, validity and reliability (APS 2000). As mentioned in Chapter 4, scientifically rigorous approaches certainly can add much to knowledge base, confidence and safeguard the interests of the client groups they serve, but too much attachment as "one that knows" may lead to clinical interactions with the elderly that are ageist (APS 2000). I believe that it is critical for all clinicians to be aware of the disempowering contexts that can arise – for all client populations – when therapists assume an identity as "knower" or "expert". This is a counselling principle held strongly by Narrative Therapists (Bubenzer, West and Boughner 1995; White 1992).

Is it possible that strong interests in measurement – to know with certainty – could make it harder to embrace what is not easily measurable and to adopt a more curious "don't know" stance? A stance that is comfortable being open to however the client wishes to frame their situation instead of one saturated with the dominant values of mainstream psychology? In the studies that have asserted the success of particular interventions with older clientele, how many have involved wary 92-year-olds of "the lucky generation" who are bed bound, not feeling themselves, but also not interested in being defined as one with a disorder – or even as having a problem? If this is not the case, then how representative are the outcomes of these studies for the oldest old living in care?

Could being senior friendly be unwittingly sabotaged by making judgements about what is wrong and having preconceived ideas about how to "fix" a problem? By determinedly believing in a set of processes that science tells us will work – and by speaking about efficacy of intervention as if it relates to all the sub-groups of those 65 and over? In this instance, where is the room for practices that allow the client to be the expert, to create space for "not knowing", to explore modalities that may not have a strong evidence base but encourage in-depth exploration in meaning-making, and maybe not to even think in terms of "need" at all? Crawford and Walker (2008) suggest that when practitioners assess older adults there is a tendency to focus on "need" rather than strengths and that this could lead to forms of ageism that are constraining factors on the relationship and intervention effectiveness.

Practices that empower rather than constrict are ones that seek to understand, not judge, and acknowledge that, "of all the experts in the care of older people, the greatest experts are older people themselves" (Department of Health 2002, p.1, in Tanner and Harris 2008). Tanner and Harris (2008) go on to suggest that narrative approaches that understand how people construct their own realities can positively affect change and focus more on, "strengths and successes rather than problems and deficits" (p.143.)

A flexible and respectful practice is one that is willing to accept the client's "truth" of their situation which may or may not identify with words like "depression" or "anxiety". It also may not be a relationship where the caregiver is consulted or seen as the expert but the other way around! Perhaps the challenging of prejudices found in gerontological research and literature that the Australian Psychological Society speak of (APS 2000, p.4) could be extended to consider how mainstream psychology could – by virtue of its confidence – be blind to how advanced seniors want to be engaged and how they want to be seen and supported? Maybe they do not even want the label of "mental health" for their issues at all? Maybe values that align themselves strongly with a medical or scientific orientation need to be suspended because of the inequality they generate? The discipline of psychology has much to offer, and extends well beyond a focus on clinical populations or problems alone, but the dominant nature with which it asserts itself should be viewed with a critical eye.

Internal programme contexts

Harold has been mourning the loss of his friend Ralph, but his face lights up when you enter the room. He is not one for gushy appreciation but the "hello" that holds its gaze steady is a sign that your encounters are valued. There are more tears today but also of talk about getting out and active again – as much as his body will allow – and you gently indicate that the therapeutic relationship will soon end. "Guess that means I'm not a hopeless case then if you want to get rid of me?!" Harold says with an impish smile. It is not how you would have framed it but, yes, you agree that he has done a valiant job managing this setback and seems to be more determined to live each day as it comes and find as much meaning in it as he can. Elizabeth is spoken of again, this bringing another tear to his eye. He can't lose sight of her, he says, even if some days are bloody awful. You write his next appointment down and say goodbye.

Two weeks later the clinical nurse sees you before your rounds and comes over. "I'm sorry I should've contacted you but we've been so busy! It's Harold. He's gone – peacefully in his sleep two days ago." She adds, "It's lucky you came today. Elizabeth is pretty cut up. She's still here collecting the last of his things. We've got someone new in the room tomorrow," then with an embarrassed apology, "Sorry." No, it's okay, you say. You know how nurses need to think and, judging from this one, how she is also feeling. "He was a good sort," she says and you give each other a smile.

Elizabeth's face is pale and downcast. It does not even look like she has registered that you are in the room until, all of a sudden, she sits and sobs. You close the door and decide that, just for today, the walker will be a good enough chair. "I can't believe that he's gone." She takes a breath and looks at you with imploring intensity. "It just doesn't feel real." She is not searching for your pearls of wisdom. Your energy and attention are mostly what she needs to melt the icicles of shock and disbelief. And you know that offering this type of bereavement care – a listening ear even though the "client" has died – is likely to reduce the risk of Elizabeth experiencing complicated grief responses much later on. After an hour she is more composed. There is even a faint smile as she speaks about how supportive the bowling club have been. "Thanks," she says, "for all you've done. I know Harold benefited greatly from the time you spent with him – for how you helped both of us." Hugging is not normally an activity you encourage with clients but Elizabeth initiates it and it seems like the kind thing to do. Technically you should give her an evaluation form but really? It does not seem right and you bid her adieu. As you walk toward your car again you feel sadness but also satisfaction – the need to acknowledge a life that has ended and feeling for those left behind but also thankful that you played a part in being a comfort for Harold and his wife Elizabeth.

There is one element in this example, in the whole process of therapeutic engagement with Harold, that illuminates a road blocker to relevance in senior-friendly practice: evaluation. For those of you who are well schooled in the importance of evidence-based practices your lips might be twitching mantras about the necessity of programme evaluations for funding. This is not to say that measuring for outcomes and obtaining client feedback are irrelevant. But I would like to stress the importance of creating policy and practice models for older adults in care that are relevant and empowering.

For example, please consider the problems that might arise for people like Harold and Elizabeth if:

- Evaluation practices do not adjust for the large scale losses common in an advanced senior cohort. Even very user-friendly tools like the Emotion Thermometers have their limitation when used to measure therapy effectiveness because while circumstances might have sent mood spiralling down again (a good friend dies), therapy could still be very much appreciated and helpful. And then there is the possibility that illness or death prevents the clinician from obtaining any outcome at all.

- Evaluation practices rely heavily on quantitative pre/post measures like the Geriatric Depression Scale which may not adequately capture distress or improvement, may not always be relevant if depressive symptoms are not the feature, may not be an empowering pre/post measure for "the lucky generation" because of the focus on pathology and may be too demanding to complete for those with very complex and co-morbid presentations.

- Evaluation practices do not customize client feedback tools used in other programmes (with a much younger clientele) to cater for the unique needs of older adults. What if they cannot see or write or post the form back and require the clinician to fill it out for them – hardly comfortable if they have negative feedback to offer? And what if the questions are too difficult, or too many, for this population group to answer?

- Evaluation practices do not place a premium on qualitative measures such as semi-structured interview questions (recorded and then transcribed for funding bodies) that are as much a chance to review therapy outcomes as they are to consider the senior's experience of the programme. Supplementing an individual focus on therapy outcomes with one that seeks to understand how the programme is being experienced can prevent other disempowering contexts. For example, where decline is occurring at a rapid pace and scores of distress are still high, the client can feel like they are being the one evaluated and not the programme. Evaluation practices should have a broad definition of "client" so that, if the original client dies, then significant others can be included in bereavement care and consulted as part of programme feedback.

I am no research or evaluation guru. Perhaps others more clever than me can solve these conundrums. I would welcome this to be investigated because work with older adults in care is even more specialized than a palliative care context which shares some of the aforementioned complexities. Therefore, programme policy and practice frameworks need to consider the unique needs and challenges of catering to an older adult clientele – especially with regard to evaluation. Beneficence is again relevant here to ensure that internal programmes are designed and implemented in a way that upholds dignity and are not unwittingly ageist or unhelpful by focusing too much on outcomes.

The Australian Psychological Society suggested that ageist attitudes are present when seniors are "seen as failures of the system because they deny health professionals the achievement of the much sought after goal of a cure" (APS 2000 p.4). I suspect that ageism is also present when psychological services for older adults have the same expectations of "cure" or "outcomes" as other programmes with much younger clients. Relevancy, it would seem, is best achieved in not just tailoring psychological approaches to an older clientele but in having stand-alone specialist programmes that live and breathe all the determinants needed to be senior friendly: specialist clinics or organizations that are dotted around every city and house within them psychotherapists from a range of disciplines, as well as medical and other allied staff, who provide centre-based and mobile consulting. True, some countries are more advanced in providing this than others, but with Boomers set to increase in years and service demand, offering such a service worldwide may become a necessity.

Finally, as an example of how useful qualitative feedback can be I would like to share with you what I learnt from a 95-year-old client the other day in our sixth session. I asked her, "So I'm wondering what this therapy thing has been like for you so far – what have you noticed or appreciated – what has it meant for you?" Her response:

Well, I can't quite tell you how things are different but I feel different. I feel better about myself and I think I've accepted more being here. I was telling my daughter the other day that I wasn't too sure about this service that you were offering. I didn't think it would do anything. I've always managed perfectly well – I've got by! I was taught that you just "got on with things". I didn't think that talking about things would do much for me. But I do feel more relief and you've helped me see that I'm not weak for feeling the way I do. Do you know – now I even don't mind the idea of going on with life.

Her feedback reminded me of Mary whom you were introduced to in the Preface. However, where Mary had rather astounding pre/post scores on the Geriatric Depression Scale (GDS), the same could not be said for this lady – not even on the Emotion Thermometers measure. For example, at our initial session, overall distress was rated 5 out of 10, sadness 5 out of 10, and frustration 9 out of 10. At session six her rating for overall distress was 7 out of 10, for sadness it was 8 out of 10, and she scored frustration 9 out of 10. Furthermore her score for the GDS at our initial session was 9 out of 15 and this only went down one point at session six. What needs to be considered, here, is that since our initial session her eyesight has diminished considerably making it impossible now for her to both read and sew (much loved pastimes) and recently there has been a death in her family.

However, as her verbal feedback suggests, her "mindset" seems to have improved considerably. Imagine if quantitative data was solely relied on or supplemented by an ineffective client survey form? The "feedback gold" that my client offered is extremely important, I believe, for internal programme contexts to value and capture. But if the funding bodies that support such programmes are ignorant about the need to resist a "one size fits all" approach to policy and practice then it makes it harder for internal programme contexts to be senior friendly. A constraint at one system level can have a flow-down effect. This is why relevant programmes of specialist care need to be valued at all system levels. And this is no more the case than at the highest system level: with external socio-political contexts.

External socio-political contexts

Looking more broadly it is perhaps not surprising that models of psychological services, and the organizations that supply them, are influenced by the socio-political contexts that surround them. If governments locally and nationally are committed to valuing seniors then service delivery models will reflect a rich diversity about how health – including mental health – can be promoted and sustained. Careful attention needs to be paid to what agendas are being promoted – if service delivery models serve the agendas of agencies more than their clients (APS 2000; Tanner and Harris 2008) – or are limited by virtue of ignorance about the psychological and emotional needs of older people, especially of those in care.

Even the notion of "mental health" might need to be understood better. It is intriguing indeed that definitions of "mental health" still do not seem to allow for sub-clinical experiences of distress – or at least grief-related clinical depression – that are so common for older adults. As an example, in my country both a Social Work position paper (AASW 2014) and a local government health framework policy for older adults (Government of South Australia 2009) limit mental health definitions to issues of a psychiatric or chronic nature and not the breadth of distress that the APS (2000) refer to, especially in relation to life transitions common for this cohort. External socio-political contexts need to be awake to the multi-faceted psychological and emotional needs that face older adults – especially the oldest old – and be interested in applying positive ageing principles across all areas of wellbeing.

Accessibility all round

Being senior friendly is to be accessible – in every conceivable way: from the language you use that conveys respect for how an advanced senior understands their world to active interests in successful ageing across all institutions of society. Ageism can affect how governments allocate resources, how attractive work with older adults is, and even how eligible seniors themselves feel about accessing services.

The following provides four recommendations, a policy platform if you like, that I believe would create more accessible options for senior psychological health: private rebates that appreciate complexity, models of training and practice not dominated by clinical psychology, services free from requiring a mental health care plan and active attempts to offset internalized ageism. I appreciate that there might be variances with how relevant these solutions are to you depending on which country you live in – but I hope that the sentiment behind these suggestions can still be relevant for policy and practice worldwide.

Private rebates that appreciate complexity

I invite you to think over all that you have learnt of Harold and Elizabeth's experience of counselling and the sort of therapy context you were encouraged to imagine. Let us recap: you had multiple interactions with care staff at the facility, you perhaps also needed to contact Harold's medical practitioner in the beginning with the GDS score and request a medication review, in the beginning there was a strong possibility that Harold was going to send you packing out the door within the first five minutes, and there were interruptions from facility staff that extended the time needed for a session. Of course, there was also the time that you visited only to discover that Harold had died and that Elizabeth was the one in need. In addition there could have been times when other relatives wanted to contact you, times where Harold was too unwell for a session or hospitalized, or personal needs he had to attend to making session length go over time.

At the time of writing, in my country of Australia, there is currently an urgent call for our Medicare system[23] to expand its criteria so that private practitioners can provide mental health services to pensioners of government-funded long-term care facilities. This is a welcome move and would make it more possible for a plethora of older adults to have access to psychotherapeutic intervention – because there are a dismal number of government-funded programmes offering this or systems of care that fund facility-based counsellors. But my concern is that even if the likes of Medicare made consulting in facilities possible then in *all* of the situations above related to Harold, the practitioner would not have been able to make a claim. They would not have been paid for their effort.

Yes, practices like phoning before you visit could reduce inconveniences (if the resident has a phone or you do not get an agency nurse) but the fact remains that work with older adults means an increased likelihood of session cancellation due to a host of variables *and* the need to liaise regularly with multiple parties. How attractive is it for practitioners to be engaged in this work and would disinterest affect how accessible psychological services are for advanced seniors? If governments are interested in healthy ageing then rebate models need to appreciate the complexities of delivering services to older adults so that practitioners do not just sigh and say, "Too hard!"

Models of training and practice not dominated by clinical psychology

As I have suggested before, the discipline of psychology, in its many forms, offers much. However, I have also referred to mindsets, values and practices that could limit effective practice with seniors. It is not my intention here to denigrate my colleagues in psychological practice but merely to point out the virtues of diversity of orientation when it comes to setting the standard and working with advanced seniors. Other professions, like mental health social workers, also have interest and skill in working psychotherapeutically with seniors.

For example, in tabling the range of contribution social workers can have in age care the Scope of Social Work in Aged Care 2015 (AASW 2015) paper identifies counselling related to grief, loss, adjustment to illness, transition to residential care, palliative care and interfamily relationships (p.5). All are issues that qualified practitioners in this profession can ably manage. Accessibility in this context encourages a range of voices to emerge in training, practice and management opportunities related to psychological services for older adults.

A visit to the recently established My Aged Care website is a case in point. The only option related to counselling in the "Allied Health and Therapy Services" is "Psychologist". No "Mental Health Social Worker" and certainly not recognition of a specialist counsellor under the title "Gerontological Psychotherapist". Counsellors from a range of backgrounds and disciplines have, I believe, much to offer the aged care sector and confidence should not be restricted to the definitions of best practice as set by the field of geropsychology.

Services free from requiring a mental health care plan

Over the years I have had the benefit of experiencing the difference between working with older adults in both specialist programmes and in private practice. Unlike most other psychological services – delivered through an organization or privately – these specialist programmes have not required that referrals relate to a mental health care plan from a medical practitioner, standard for accessing a subsidized or free service in Australia. What a blessing. Very few advanced seniors that I have come in contact with, especially in a residential setting, would have agreed to accepting – let alone requested – a psychological service. And yet these same seniors, after being consulted in a sensitive way, have gone on to be actively engaged in the therapeutic process and reaped many rewards for doing so. Also not needing a mental health care plan makes the whole process of assessing for interest and suitability easier. It allows the psychotherapist who is familiar with both a senior friendly "spiel" and is aware of the range of factors that will inhibit or advance psychotherapeutic engagement to triage a referral and decide if it is amenable to a more formal approach or requires referral to another agency.

Active attempts to offset internalized ageism

Internalized ageism can prevent seniors from believing that their needs are worth the attention – that they are worth the effort (APS 2000; Hitchcock 2015; Tanner and Harris 2008). This, coupled with a generational discomfort with entitlement or emotional issues, can have the current cohort of advanced seniors extremely reluctant to access psychological services and also to be associated with anything related to "mental". Programmes that are gentle in engagement and explanation of service give room for seniors to "try before they buy". Public campaigns could also raise general awareness, and specifically target seniors, in the benefits of seeking a psychological service for distress late in life. Television would be the perfect avenue for awareness through advertisements given how much seniors seem to watch it.

Consult below and advocate up

Being senior friendly is about being awake to disempowering contexts that inhibit the effective provision of mental health services to older people in care. This work is consultative and political. It requires practitioners, managers, funding bodies, policy advisors and politicians to listen to and value the voice of seniors and agitate for change where necessary. At every system level, opportunities can be found to build psychotherapeutic programmes that are relevant and sensitive to the unique needs of an older adult clientele. No context is immune from ageism. Even in the private space of counselling, disempowering attitudes can infiltrate and choke like smoke, be perpetuated either implicitly or explicitly. As a mental health social worker my commitment to creating empowering contexts runs deep. I am a social worker before I am a psychotherapist. It seems perfectly natural to me to examine systems at all levels and "advocate up". My profession's Code of Ethics demands such a commitment. It states that:

> Social work aims to maximise the development of human potential and the fulfilment of human needs by...working to address and redress inequity and injustice...working to achieve human rights and social justice through social development, social and systemic change, advocacy and the ethical conduct of research. (Australian Association of Social Workers 2010, p.7)
>
> [The social work profession also] respects the inherent dignity, worth and autonomy of every person [and the] human rights of individuals and groups. (p.12)

We must not accept the status quo if it is at odds with a senior-friendly practice. At every system level – from the micro to the macro – we can consult below and advocate up. We can learn what is important to seniors and how they would like to be defined. We can challenge ageism by calling for systemic change. And, as the final section suggests, we can "bring sexy back" in how we think about and engage older adults.

Bring sexy back!

It is understandable if you are struggling to reconcile images of a smooth moving Justin Timberlake singing, "I'm bringing sexy back..." with the experience of working in aged care! Sexy is often everything that aged care is not. But by using the word "sexy" I am not referring to the high octane experience of being intimate with someone. Who knows though, your older adult clients may well want to talk about such things! How senior friendly to encourage this! What I am referring to is bringing the spice or pizzazz associated with respect back to our Western society that appears to have lost its way in valuing seniors.

Let me ask you something. How do you feel if someone asks for your opinion? You know, for something really important that you have a vested interest in? Is it possible that you might feel appreciated? A little flushed with satisfaction that your opinion matters and that someone is taking an interest in *you*? Is not that what sexy is about? Your mind and body soaring when you know your hold on another's affections? Turning the heat up might not just relate to your physical world but also your sense of value. If we equate "sexy" with value and appeal then how might we bring sexy back in our view of advanced seniors – in our practice of psychotherapy with them? While we may no longer be a tribal culture where elders have a strong role and are included in the community, how can psychotherapeutic intervention contribute to a reclaiming of senior status and an interest in consulting them?

In 1971 American anthropologist the late Barbara Myerhoff began a study of an immigrant Jewish community in Venice, California who were in their 80s and 90s. It was part of a wider investigation into ethnicity and ageing and resulted in an award-winning documentary entitled *Number Our Days* (Myerhoff 1976). Reflecting on her interactions with these elderly Jewish people, Barbara was struck by the degree to which they felt invisible and how, "Among very old people…they may come to doubt not only their worth and potency, not only their value, but the very fact of their existence" (Myerhoff 1986, p.265).

I remember my own impressions as I began consulting advanced seniors in 2009. I, too, was struck by stories that related to invisibility and of how many related to this exact term as they opened up about experiences of isolation and feeling forgotten – the forgotten generation. You may remember that in the introduction I referred to a woman who, only very recently, described her experience as feeling "thrown away". It is the experience that Doctor Karen Hitchcock (2015) illuminates in her impassioned essay "Dear Life" referred to earlier. And, with regard to the ageist attitudes in Chapter 8, it can also relate to feeling unattractive, obsolete, not worth it, hopeless and inadequate when life goes against an embodiment of "progress" which society prizes with such vigour.

Where is the sense of value in this? Of appeal? But what Barbara also discovered in her interactions with this Jewish community was the significance of witnessing their various expressions of personal and collective identity. She reflected that when cultural groups perform ceremonies or rituals:

> They tell stories, comment, portray, and mirror… Such performances are opportunities for appearing, an indispensable ingredient of being itself, for unless we exist in the eyes of others, we may come to doubt

even our own existence. Being is a social, psychological construct, made, not given. Thus it is erroneous to think of performance as optional, arbitrary, or merely decorative embellishments as we in Western societies are inclined to do. In this sense, arenas for appearing are essential, and culture serves as a stage as well as mirror, providing opportunities for self and collective proclamations of being. (Myerhoff 1982, pp.103–104)

How does this relate to psychotherapy with seniors? The link Barbara made with these observations and her experiences with people in this elderly community was that through the process of performing, of engaging in what she called "definitional ceremony", these seniors not only felt visible but were able to sharpen how they defined themselves. Moreover, she suggested that:

Definitional ceremonies deal with the problems of invisibility and marginality; they are strategies that provide opportunities for being seen and in one's own terms, garnering witness to one's worth, vitality, and being. (Myerhoff 1986, p.267)

This is what counselling can offer: a format that exhibits and also reflects back essential elements of one's being. From this viewpoint, practices like Reminiscence Therapy can become more than just a distraction or even of establishing greater meaning for seniors. The very process of it can facilitate visibility and a strengthening of the historical self. Not only this but being invited to tell – to perform and be visible – can be highly significant. Barbara offers this:

A story told aloud to progeny or peers is, of course, more than text. It is an event. When it is done properly, presentationally, its effect on the listener is profound, and the latter is more than a mere passive receiver or validator. The listener is changed. (Myerhoff 1986, p. 116)

This is exactly what led to the development of the Life Story Interview mentioned in Chapter 5. It was an attempt to respond to how advanced seniors seemed to want to give and, in that, strengthen their own agenda, self-definition and worth as they hear how a witness is impacted by their story. What greater gift is there to give someone than for them to know that they matter, that they have an effect, and that they can be seen?

When we bring "sexy back" to the counselling context with seniors we open ourselves up to being a recipient and not just a giver or helper. We allow ourselves to be taught, to let an older adult tell their story and be witness to their version of "truth" without interpreting it, diagnosing it or challenging anything other than what they themselves want to challenge. We let them change us and, in doing so, enable an awakening of more helpful self-understanding of how they want to know themselves and who they know themselves to be.

Being senior friendly is enabling identities not limited to "depressed", "anxious" or "disordered". In the tenets of positive ageing it means moving away from definitions that refer to "deficits", "pathology" and "frailty". It moves toward an inclusive stance, valuing social capital and encouraging opportunities for participation (Lui, Warbuton and Winterton 2011, p. 276). Being senior friendly and bringing sexy back is not merely – and maybe not even – following a scientifically approved set of processes. It is, as Chapter 6 suggested, to forget about the dance routine for a while and just move to the music. To free yourself from the cobwebs of agenda and just relax into your interest of this person as a human being.

Summary

Through a trilogy of elements a challenge is set: excite and equip an army of psychotherapists from a range of disciplines to respond to the psychological needs of our ageing population. While advances are noted in various countries, the fact remains that the availability of specialist counsellors in the field of aged care is a global concern.

Not only this, but a special breed of senior has been identified who warrants particular attention. Advanced seniors currently in their 80s and 90s, especially those in facility settings, are often overlooked and left unsupported in their experiences of distress. The story of Harold and his wife Elizabeth has highlighted the issues common to this age group but also how psychotherapists might effectively engage and intervene. Those of "the lucky generation" can be particularly wary about counselling. Care and sensitivity to generational nuances are needed to increase comfort and positive therapeutic outcomes not necessarily dependent on mainstream psychological practice. While distress is not inevitable for the advanced senior cohort, understanding the variety of ways in which wellbeing can be affected is essential as is ability to work within an aged care facility context.

Assessment was also cited as an important consideration but distinction was made between informal and formal assessment. Related to the importance of informal assessment was implicit therapeutic work which preferred a biographical and exploratory entry point over one framed by deficit and an explicit helper role. Along with assessment was a whole smorgasbord of issues common to those late in life as well as management strategies and a unique integrated model of intervention.

In Part 3, attention was given to bigger picture issues: the care needs of you, the psychotherapist, and socio-ethical-political contexts. Specifically, five ageist attitudes were identified and broader contexts of practice were discussed that psychotherapists need to be alert to in their work with older adults. Furthermore, a senior-friendly approach was encouraged and seen to relate to four main domains: initial engagement approach, intervention and relationship, internal programme contexts, and external socio-political contexts. Integral to adopting senior-friendly protocols at a variety of system levels, this was discussed in relation to the notions of accessibility. In particular, accessibility was believed to be promoted if four conditions were apparent: private rebates that appreciate complexity, models of training and practice not dominated by clinical psychology, services free from requiring a mental health care plan, and active attempts to offset internalized ageism. Social work ethics and values were then identified and linked to a multi-systemic practice that "consults down" and "advocates up".

Collectively, being senior friendly related to an interest in a senior's story. In the introduction I shared my own story about how I came to work therapeutically with seniors. With no formal training in the field of geropsychology, but years of experience as a counsellor, I explained how my colleague and I set out to learn as best we could how to work in this brand new programme. Despite often feeling uncertain it was the seniors whom we consulted that taught us all we needed to know. They are the voices that told me what mattered.

The Insight Meditation Center in California share on their website about a "beginner's mind" and how this state of "not-knowing" is highly valued. The description is an adaptation of a talk (Fronsdal 2004) and goes on to say:

An expert may know a subject deeply, yet be blinded to new possibilities by his or her preconceived ideas. In contrast, a beginner may see with fresh, unbiased eyes. The practice of beginner's mind is to cultivate an ability to meet life without preconceived ideas, interpretations, or judgments.

I believe that work with seniors needs to be like this: meeting every person and situation anew, just as American poet Mary Oliver suggests making room for the unimaginable (2010). Connect. Listen. Let older adults teach you about what life was, is for them now, and all that is important. You never know what you might learn.

The End

APPENDICES

Appendix 1

Determining Suitability and Tailoring Intervention

Working with Older Adults in Care

Below is intended as a form of reflective practice and is an informal assessment tool. It is not intended to be used with the client and is not a validated assessment measure. It is for the counsellor's private use to better determine suitability and, if relevant, consider how they might proceed. Please note that as older adults in care can fluctuate considerably during the course of therapy this sheet may also be used at various stages of therapy.

Instructions: simply insert your rating in the right hand column as either a scale of 0–10 or as low, medium, high, or unsure.

Main measure	Sub measure		Rating
Motivation to change/take responsibility			
Ability to change?			
How much of the problem is their problem?			
How much is it someone else's, i.e. staff, family, other resident, GP?			
Engagement or interest in contact?			
Ability to engage?	Sight?		
	Cognitive?	Memory?	
		Insight?	
		Comprehension?	
	Hearing?		
	Hand mobility?		
	Pain/discomfort?		
	Environment?	Privacy?	
		Noise?	
		Interruption?	
Familiarity with counselling process/expectations?			
Complexity and severity of issues?			
Level of outside support?			
Level of concern re: privacy/stigma?			
Level of comfort re: discussing personals?			

Appendix 2

Intake and First Few Sessions

Working with Older Adults in Care

1	Have you seen a counsellor before? (note experience if yes)	Yes ☐	No ☐
2	It's common for seniors to experience the following. Which of the following do you relate to?		
	2.1 Missing your pets (name of pet/s)	Yes ☐	No ☐
	2.2 Having frequent bouts of teariness or sadness	Yes ☐	No ☐
	2.3 Feeling lonely	Yes ☐	No ☐
	2.4 Feeling a loss of privacy and control	Yes ☐	No ☐
	2.5 Losing some function in your body that bothers you	Yes ☐	No ☐
	2.6 Being in a lot of pain or discomfort	Yes ☐	No ☐
	2.7 Forgetting important things often	Yes ☐	No ☐
	2.8 Having thoughts about death or dying	Yes ☐	No ☐
	2.9 Feeling isolated from family or friends	Yes ☐	No ☐
	2.10 Being bothered by a loss of independence	Yes ☐	No ☐
	2.11 Grieving the loss or decline of your spouse	Yes ☐	No ☐
	2.12 Feeling like you have lost a sense of identity or purpose	Yes ☐	No ☐
	2.13 Missing your old life prior to moving into this ACF	Yes ☐	No ☐
	2.14 Lived or served in a war zone	Yes ☐	No ☐
3	What things, people or situations are bothering you most at the moment?		
4	How have you overcome difficult periods in your life?		
5	What gives you joy or makes you feel good? Are there any memories that do this?		
6	Genogram and key family members/historical events		

Appendix 3

Some Experiences of Grief

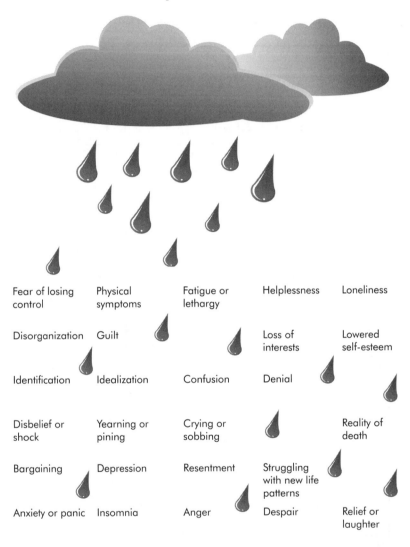

Fear of losing control	Physical symptoms	Fatigue or lethargy	Helplessness	Loneliness
Disorganization	Guilt		Loss of interests	Lowered self-esteem
Identification	Idealization	Confusion	Denial	
Disbelief or shock	Yearning or pining	Crying or sobbing		Reality of death
Bargaining	Depression	Resentment	Struggling with new life patterns	
Anxiety or panic	Insomnia	Anger	Despair	Relief or laughter

Felicity Chapman: www.yourstoryline.com.au

This is a modified version of the Northern Metropolitan Community Health Service handout, 2004.

Definitions

Advanced senior
Relates to the "oldest old" – those who are 85 years or older. Both the term "advanced" and "senior" have positive associations, particularly in the world of education and employment. I like the idea of using terms that have positive associations with a group of people who can often feel redundant and lacking in status – particularly in Western societies.

Acceptance and Commitment Therapy
Acceptance and Commitment Therapy is a "third wave" psychotherapeutic intervention which uses mindfulness-based practices to enable people to be present and open up to unpleasant experiences while moving toward valued living. Foundational tenets include: acceptance, defusion, observer self, mindfulness, values and committed action.

Aged care facility (related terms: long-term care facility, nursing home, residential care facility)
An aged care facility is a place of long-term care for those with medium to high care needs and/or for those with palliative care needs or are advanced in years. They are places where a variety of professionals attend to the wellbeing of residents: care attendants, enrolled nurses, registered nurses, clinical care managers, occupational therapists, physiotherapists, podiatrists, Lifestyle staff, kitchen staff, cleaning staff, doctors, and management – and visiting businesses or specialists.

Ageism
Ageism is stereotyping and discriminating against individuals or groups on the basis of their age and was coined in 1969 by Doctor Robert Butler. Butler defined "ageism" as a combination of three connected elements: any prejudice against the ageing process or older people, discrimination against older people, and practices or policies that reinforce negative stereotypes.

Alzheimer's disease

Alzheimer's disease is the most common form of dementia. It can affect adults at any age, but usually occurs after age 65. Familial Alzheimer's disease is a very rare genetic condition and means that the person will develop Alzheimer's at a very young age: 40s or 50s.

Attachment theory

Attachment theory is based on the pioneering work of John Bowlby and his belief that an infant needs to develop a relationship with at least one primary caregiver for the child's successful social and emotional development, and in particular for learning how to effectively regulate their feelings.

Beneficence

Beneficence is a concept used mainly in research ethics. It emphasizes the importance of the welfare of any research participant and strongly opposes any action or inaction that might be considered maleficence – practice which opposes the welfare of any research participant.

Clinical social worker or mental health social worker

Clinical social workers address individual and family problems such as serious illness, substance abuse and domestic conflict. Work typically encompasses evidence-based counselling or psychotherapy and client engagement practices are often similar, or identical, to those of a registered psychologist. Qualifications reflect the specialist nature of this role as practitioners have additional clinical training, usually a master's degree, to supplement their undergraduate social work degree.

Cognitive Behavioural Therapy

Cognitive Behavioural Therapy is a psychosocial intervention based on the belief that thought distortions and maladaptive behaviours play a role in the development and maintenance of psychological disorders, and that symptoms and associated distress can be reduced by teaching new information-processing skills and coping mechanisms. Intervention focuses on solving current problems and changing unhelpful patterns in cognitions (e.g. thoughts, beliefs and attitudes), behaviours and emotional experiences. A foundational tenet is that of cognitive reappraisal.

Compassion fatigue

Compassion fatigue is common in paid or unpaid endeavours which bring the person in close contact with caring roles or with people experiencing distress. Those affected can be health professionals such as nurses, psychotherapists and doctors; crisis intervention workers such as policemen and paramedics; and long-term support people such as friends, family and members of the clergy. It is characterized by a gradual reduction of compassion over time and is also known as Secondary Traumatic Stress.

Compassion satisfaction

"Compassion satisfaction" and "compassion fatigue" are two sides of the same coin. Both relate to paid or unpaid acts of service. But where compassion fatigue relates to a sense of depletion, compassion satisfaction relates to a sense of fullness or completion. The context or the person toward whom an act of service is directed fulfils a need in the "giver" – usually in an altruistic way or where the act of service is very consistent with the giver's value set.

Counsellor

A counsellor is similar to a psychotherapist except that their level of involvement is more short term and focused on present issues that are easily resolved on the conscious level. Examples include study or work stress, worry, relationship tension, grief and distress related to life transition/opportunities. A counsellor (like other psychotherapists or clinicians) aims to develop a strong therapeutic alliance, assess for risk, and use reflective listening skills and client-centred strategies to bring about relief and change in relation to practical or immediate issues. Counsellors usually have diploma-level qualifications.

Dementia

The most common type of dementia is Alzheimer's disease. Dementia is a broad category of brain diseases that cause a long-term and often gradual decrease in the ability to think and remember that is great enough to affect a person's daily functioning. Other common types include vascular dementia, Lewy body dementia and frontotemporal dementia.

Dignity Therapy

Dignity Therapy was developed by Doctor Harvey Chochinov to assist people dealing with end of life issues. The intervention is brief – typically just a 30- to 60-minute session – in which questions are asked that encourage the dying patient to reflect on what their life has meant to them and what legacies they would like to leave behind. The conversation is recorded, transcribed, edited and then returned within a few days to the patient, who is given the opportunity to read the transcript and make changes before a final version is produced. Many choose to share the document with family and friends.

Dysphoria

Dysphoria is a profound state of unease or dissatisfaction. It may also be linked with depression, anxiety or agitation.

Frontotemporal dementia

Frontotemporal dementia is the name given to dementia when it is due to progressive damage to the frontal and/or temporal lobes of the brain. The right and left frontal lobes at the front of the brain are involved in mood, social behaviour, attention, judgement, planning and self-control. Damage can lead to reduced intellectual abilities and changes in personality, emotion and behaviour. The right and left temporal lobes at the two sides of the brain are involved in processing what we hear and understanding what we hear and see. Damage may lead to difficulty recognizing objects or understanding or expressing language.

Geriatric Depression Scale

In the Geriatric Depression Scale, questions are answered "yes" or "no". The GDS is commonly used as a routine part of a comprehensive geriatric assessment. One point is assigned to each answer and the cumulative score is rated on a scoring grid. The grid sets a range of 0–9 as "normal", 10–19 as "mildly depressed" and 20–30 as "severely depressed". A diagnosis of clinical depression should not be based on GDS results alone.

Gerontology

Gerontology is the study of the biological, social, cultural, cognitive and psychological aspects of ageing. It is not the same as geriatrics, which is the branch of medicine that specializes in the treatment of existing disease in older adults. Gerontologists include researchers and practitioners in the fields of biology, nursing, medicine, criminology, dentistry, social work, physical and occupational therapy, psychiatry, psychology, sociology, economics, political science, architecture, geography, pharmacy, public health, housing and anthropology.

Geropsychology or clinical geropsychology

Professional geropsychology or clinical geropsychology is a specialty in professional psychology that applies the knowledge and methods of psychology to understand and help older people and their families to maintain wellbeing, overcome problems and achieve quality of life. Clinical geropsychologists work with professionals across medical and health care disciplines and perform psychotherapy and psychological evaluations. It was recognized as a specialty area by the American Psychological Association in 2010.

Gerontological psychotherapist

This is a term I have devised to denote any psychotherapy practitioner who specializes in work with older adults – in particular older adults who are advanced in years and who are living in long-term care – and who is not a qualified geropsychologist. Occupations included in this category: psychologists, mental health social workers, mental health occupational therapists, mental health nurses and qualified counsellors/psychotherapists.

Hypo-arousal or hyper-arousal

Arousal refers to the physiological state of readiness or general state of excitation of one's nervous system. Arousal states lie on a continuum from low to high, and the ability to maintain optimal arousal levels is often required for adaptive interaction with one's environment. Hypo-arousal refers to insufficient nervous system activation; for example, lethargy or inattention. Hyper-arousal refers to too much nervous system activation; for example, flushed face or exaggerated startle responses.

Kessler Psychological Distress Scale

The Kessler Psychological Distress Scale (K10) consists of ten questions about the level of anxiety and depressive symptoms a person may have experienced in the most recent four-week period.

Lewy body dementia

Lewy body disease is caused by the degeneration and death of nerve cells in the brain. The name comes from the presence of abnormal spherical structures, called Lewy bodies, which develop inside nerve cells. It is thought that these may contribute to the death of brain cells.

Limbic system

The limbic system serves many functions. It helps control affects/emotions, memory, sensory processing, time perception, attention, consciousness, instincts, autonomic/vegetative control, and actions/motor behaviour.

Life Review

Erikson's Theory of Psychosocial Development, combined with Doctor Robert Butler's definition of reminiscence, formed the blueprint for structured Life Review and gave way to the Life Review and Experiencing Form developed by Doctor Barbara Haight in 1982. Its aim is to reduce depression, increase life satisfaction, self-acceptance, bonding, catharsis and reconnection with significant others. Unlike other forms of reminiscence therapy, structured life review is conducted on an individual basis and involves only the reviewer and the therapeutic listener. Participants reflect on both the positive and negative aspects of their lives, evaluating the significance of these events and working through unresolved conflicts.

Maleficence

The act of committing harm.

Mental health care plan or mental health treatment plan

In Australia this relates to an assessment that a general practitioner performs which is also used as a referral for an accredited mental health professional to proceed by offering a course of treatment or number of sessions. Whether the professional is working in a private practice or for an organization, the completion of a "mental health care plan" is essential if the client is to receive a free or subsidized service through either Medicare (the federal health care system) or a government-funded agency.

Mindfulness

The term "mindfulness" is a process which cultivates a special type of awareness of present moment experiences: noticing the neutral, not grasping at the pleasant and not "fighting" with the unpleasant. While changed states might occur with the practice of mindfulness, the practice is not about trying to change states or trying to control anything. It is simply to notice all the internal and external events of the here and now. Mindfulness is a translation of the Pali term *sati* and is one element of The Noble Eightfold Path in Buddhism – the other seven being right view, right resolve, right speech, right conduct, right livelihood, right effort and right "samadhi" or meditative concentration. Mindfulness has gained significant popularity in the last few decades, largely through the work of Jon Kabat-Zinn and his Mindfulness Based Stress Reduction programme, and research is supporting its use as an effective psychological tool for the management of psychological distress.

Mindfulness-based interventions (related term: mindfulness-based practices)

Mindfulness-based interventions are therapeutic approaches that use mindfulness. The most common approaches that use mindfulness are: Mindfulness-Based Stress Reduction (MBSR), Mindfulness-Based Cognitive Therapy (MBCT), Dialectal Behaviour Therapy (DBT) and Acceptance and Commitment Therapy (ACT), all of which deliberately focus a person's attention on the present experience in a way that is non-judgemental. The efficacy of these practices is growing – especially as it relates to relapse prevention for depression, neuroplasticity, trauma management and managing pain and stress.

Narrative Therapy

Narrative Therapy is a form of psychotherapy that encourages people to arrive at their own definition of the problem and to draw on their multi-storied lives and knowledges to find alternative solutions and healing. Therapists co-author new narratives with the client by being "decentred and influential" and understanding the interplay between the "personal and the professional"; in this way therapists acknowledge how their own culture and history could negatively affect therapeutic effectiveness and actively seek to keep as their focus the client's agenda. Through this transparent and consultative process therapists also assist clients in challenging dominant discourses – social injustices – or desconstructing "truths" that are contributing to the problem in the person's life. This approach was developed during the 1970s and 1980s, largely by South Australian social worker Michael White and David Epston of New Zealand.

Positive ageing (related term: healthy ageing, ageing well, successful ageing)

Positive ageing is the process of maintaining a positive attitude, feeling good about yourself, keeping fit and healthy, and engaging fully in life as you progress in age. Positive ageing is also an acknowledgement of how unhelpful mental states (beliefs, thoughts, ideas, attitudes) can have a negative impact on physical and emotional wellbeing. Positive ageing understands that the "mind" can have a big impact on our physical and emotional wellbeing and promotes quality of life at any age.

Positive psychology

Positive psychology is the scientific study of the strengths that enable individuals and communities to thrive. The field is founded on the belief that people want to lead meaningful and fulfilling lives, to cultivate what is best within themselves, and to enhance their experiences of love, work and play. Doctor Martin Seligman is a pioneer of positive psychology (the term itself was coined by Abraham Maslow), not simply because he has a systematic theory about why happy people are happy, but because he uses the scientific method to explore it.

Psychiatrist

A psychiatrist is a physician who specializes in psychiatry, the branch of medicine focused on diagnosing, preventing, studying and treating mental disorders. Psychiatrists are medical doctors, unlike psychologists, and evaluate people to determine whether their symptoms are the result of a physical illness, a combination of physical and mental problems, or strictly psychiatric.

Psychogeriatrician

A psychiatrist subspecializing in the assessment and treatment of elderly people.

Psychologist

A psychologist is a professional who evaluates and studies mental processes and behaviour. There are many types of psychologists as reflected by the 56 divisions of the American Psychological Association (APA), but psychologists generally fall into two groups: applied and research-orientated. In the applied setting, one of the more common types is the clinical psychologist, who evaluates and treats people experiencing psychosocial problems.

Psychosis

Psychosis is a mental disorder where a person loses the capacity to be in contact with reality. They may believe or sense things that are not real and become confused or slow in their thinking. Psychosis often occurs as a part of other mental illness and features in the American Psychiatric Association's Diagnostic and Statistical Manual of Mental Disorders (DSM-5) which offers internationally recognized standard criteria for classifying mental "disorders".

Psychotherapist

A psychotherapist is similar to a counsellor except that their level of involvement is longer term and focused on helping a person understand his/her life in a profound and reflective manner. The process of psychotherapy is like "peeling away onion layers" in that a psychotherapist's work often uncovers and manages root causes of problems such as distress related to past trauma. In this way the consideration of the time line is very broad: present issues are considered in light of historical accounts and future goals or lost dreams. A psychotherapist aims to free clients from unconscious triggers or impulses through self-awareness but only works at this deep level if the client is ready. Psychotherapist qualifications vary from diploma to doctorate levels but all have supervised training.

Reminiscence Therapy

Reminiscence Therapy is a technique often used with older adults and deliberately taps into life histories in oral and/or written forms to promote wellbeing. There are different types of reminiscence which can take place. The two main subtypes are intrapersonal and interpersonal reminiscence. Intrapersonal takes a cognitive stance and occurs individually. Interpersonal is a group-based therapy. Reminiscence can then be further broken down into three specific types which are: information, evaluation and obsessive. Evaluative reminiscence is the main type of reminiscence therapy as it is based on Doctor Robert Butler's Life Review system which involves recalling memories throughout one's entire life and sharing these stories in a therapeutic group setting.

Rogerian Psychotherapy

Rogerian Psychotherapy is also known as Person-centred Therapy, Person-centred Counselling, and Client-centred Therapy. It was developed by psychologist Carl Rogers early to mid last century and is a part of the Humanistic Psychology movement. Rogerian Psychotherapy has as its focus the whole person and a fundamental belief in human potential and that people are inherently good. The therapist's role is to intervene using "unconditional positive regard" and encourages clients to express their own capabilities and creativity on the path toward healing or self-actualization.

Social work

Social work is an academic and practice-based professional discipline that seeks to facilitate the welfare of communities, individuals, families and groups. Underpinned by theories of social science and guided by principles of social justice, rights, collective responsibility and respect for diversity, social work engages people and structures to address life challenges and enhance wellbeing. Social work tries to promote social change and grassroots empowerment of people and aids in socio-economic development, social cohesion, and liberation from abuse and oppression. A practising professional with a degree in social work is called a social worker.

The Psychogeriatric Assessment Scales

The Psychogeriatric Assessment Scales provide an assessment of the clinical changes seen in dementia and depression and are used primarily with an older adult cohort. Three dimensions are reviewed in an interview with the person: cognitive impairment, depression and stroke and a further three with a staff or family member: cognitive decline, behaviour change and stroke. The scales are suitable for application both in research and in services for older adults.

Vascular dementia

Vascular dementia is the broad term for dementia associated with problems of circulation of blood to the brain. Multi-infarct dementia is probably the most common form of vascular dementia and is caused by a number of strokes, often with symptoms that develop progressively over a period of time. The strokes cause damage to the cortex of the brain, the area associated with learning, memory and language. A person with multi-infarct dementia is likely to have better insight in the early stages than people with Alzheimer's disease, and parts of their personality may remain relatively intact for longer. Symptoms may include severe depression, mood swings and epilepsy. Memory loss may or may not be a significant symptom depending on the specific brain areas where blood flow is reduced.

Wellbeing

Wellbeing, well-being, welfare or wellness is a general term for the condition of an individual or group that relates to positive or satisfying experiences of social, economic, psychological, spiritual or physical functioning.

References

Aged Rights Advocacy Service (2017) *Mandatory Reporting: Elder Abuse and the Law.* South Australia: Aged Rights Advocacy Service. Accessed on 17/04/2017 at www. sa.agedrights.asn.au/about_us

Age UK (2017) *Briefing: Health and Care for Older People in England 2017.* London: Age UK. Accessed on 19/05/2017 at www.ageuk.org.uk/Documents/EN-GB/ For-professionals/Research/The_Health_and_Care_of_Older_People_in_ England_2016.pdf?dtrk=true

American Association for Marriage and Family Therapy. (2017) *Suicide in the Elderly.* Virginia: American Association for Marriage and Family Therapy. Accessed on 11/06/2017 at www.aamft.org/iMIS15/AAMFT/Content/Consumer_Updates/ Suicide_in_the_Elderly.aspx

American Psychological Association (2014) 'Guidelines for practice with older adults.' *American Psychologist 69,* 1, 34–65.

American Psychological Association (2017) *Guidelines for Psychological Practice with Older Adults.* Washington: American Psychological Association. Accessed on 16/04/2017 at www.apa.org/practice/guidelines/older-adults.aspx

Antle, B.J. and Regehr, C. (2003) 'Beyond individual rights and freedoms: metaethics in social work research.' *Social Work 48,* 1, 135–144.

Arch, J.J. and Craske, M.G. (2008) 'Acceptance and Commitment Therapy and Cognitive Behavioral Therapy for anxiety disorders: different treatments, similar mechanisms?' *Clinical Psychology: Science and Practice 15,* 4, 263–279.

Australian Association of Social Workers (2010) *Code of Ethics.* Canberra: Australian Association of Social Workers.

Australian Association of Social Workers (2014) *AASW Position Paper: Improving Service Responses for Older People with a Mental Health Condition.* Position Paper. Canberra: Australian Association of Social Workers.

Australian Association of Social Workers (2015) *Scope of Social Work Practice: Social Workers in Aged Care.* Victoria: Australian Association of Social Workers.

Australian Association of Social Workers (2016) Personal communication, 19 February.

Australian Psychological Society (2000) *Psychology and Ageing: A Position Paper Prepared for the Australian Psychological Society by a Working Group of the Directorate of Social Issues.* Position Paper. Melbourne: The Australian Psychological Society Ltd.

Australian Psychological Society (2011) 'Suicide prevention: professional development training.' *Populations at Risk of Suicide: Topic 3,* 1–35.

Australian Psychological Society, Occupational Therapy Australia, and Australian Association of Social Workers (2011) *CBT Fundamentals: Processes and Techniques in Cognitive Behaviour Therapy.* Training manual. Melbourne: The Australian Psychological Society Ltd.

Baker, A.E.Z. and Procter, N.G. (2015) '"You Just Lose the People You Know": Relationship Loss and Mental Illness.' *Archives of Psychiatric Nursing 29*, 96–101.

Backhouse, J. and Graham, A. (2013) 'Grandparents raising their grandchildren: acknowledging the experience of grief.' *Australian Social Work 66*, 3, 440–454.

Blando J. (2014) *Counseling Older Adults.* Abingdon: Routledge.

Blyth, F.M., March, L.M., Brnabic, A.J., Jorm, L.R., Williamson, M. and Cousins, M.J. (2001) 'Chronic pain in Australia: a prevalence study.' *Pain 89*, 2–3, 127–134.

Bytheway, B. (1995) *Ageism: Rethinking Ageing Series.* New York: McGraw-Hill.

Bodmer Lutz, A. (2014) *Learning Solution-Focused Therapy: An Illustrated Guide.* Virginia: American Psychiatric Publishing.

Bubenzer, D.L., West, J.D. and Boughner, S.R. (1995) 'The Narrative Perspective.' In M. White (ed.) *Re-authoring Lives: Interviews and Essays.* Adelaide: Dulwich Centre Publications.

Briggs Myers, I. and Myers, P.B. (1995) *Gifts Differing: Understanding Personality Type* (Reprint Ed). California: Davies-Black Publishing.

Butler, D. and Moseley, L. (2013) *Explain Pain* (2nd Ed.). Adelaide: Noigroup Publications.

Byrne, G.J.A. and Pachana, N.A. (2011) 'Development and validation of a short form of the Geriatric Anxiety Inventory – the GAI-SF.' *International Psychogeriatrics 23*,1, 125–131.

Caldwell, R.L. (2005) 'At the confluence of memory and meaning – life review with older adults and families: using Narrative Therapy and the expressive arts to re-member and re-author stories of resilience.' *The Family Journal: Counselling and Therapy for Couples and Families 13*, 2, 172–174.

CHE Behavioral Services (2017) *Company Profile.* USA: CHE Behavioral Services. Accessed on 16/04/2017 at http://cheservices.com/index.html

Chowdhry, A. (2013) *Lessons Learned From 4 Steve Jobs Quotes.* Tech. New York: Forbes Magazine. Accessed on 28/07/2017 at www.forbes.com/sites/amitchowdhry/2013/10/05/lessons-learned-from-4-steve-jobs-quotes/#6c9a08e14f69

Cook, J.M. and Wiltsey Stirman, S. (2015) 'Implementation of evidence-based treatment for PTSD.' *PTSD Research Quarterly 26*, 4, 1–9.

Commonwealth of Australia (2011a) 'Caring for older Australians.' *Productivity Commission Inquiry Report 2*, 53, v–138.

Commonwealth of Australia (2011b) *Guidelines for a Palliative Approach for Aged Care in the Community Setting: Best Practice Guidelines for the Australian Context.* Best Practice Paper. Canberra: Australian Government Department of Health and Ageing.

Commonwealth of Australia (2013) *Depression in Residential Aged Care 2008–2012.* National Inquiry. Canberra: Australian Institute of Health and Welfare.

Council on the Ageing (2017) *Sign the Petition: Nursing Home Residents Deserve Better Access to Mental Health Care.* Canberra: COTA Australia. Accessed on 16/04/2017 at http://healthforolderaustralians.org.au

Crawford, K. and Walker, J. (2008) *Social Work with Older People* (2nd Ed.). Exeter: Learning Matters Limited.

Daily Mail Australia (2012) *Nazi Horrors Revisited: The Holocaust Survivors Who Only Develop PTSD in Old Age.* United Kingdom: DMG Media. Accessed on 19/04/2017 at www.dailymail.co.uk/news/article-2157725/Nazi-horrors-revisited-The-Holocaust-survivors-develop-PTSD-old-age.html

Department of Health (2006) *Guidelines for Working with People with Challenging Behaviours in Residential Aged Care Facilities: Using Appropriate Interventions and Minimising Restraint.* Best Practice Paper. Sydney: DoH. (pages 4–5 reprinted by permission, NSW Ministry of Health © 2017).

Dignity in Care (2016) *Questions Asked during Dignity Therapy.* Dignity Model and Dignity Therapy by Dr Chochinov. Canada: Manitoba Palliative Care Research Unit. Accessed on 31/05/2017 at http://dignityincare.ca/en/toolkit.html#Dignity_Therapy_ questions

Doka, K.J. (1989) *Disenfranchised Grief: Recognizing Hidden Sorrow.* New York: Lexington Books.

Dulwich Centre Publications (1999) *Narrative Therapy and Community Work: A Conference Collection.* Adelaide: Dulwich Centre Publications.

Fella, A. (2009) *Buddhism 101: Part 1.* Transcription. California: Insight Meditation Center. Accessed on 06/05/2017 at www.insightmeditationcenter.org/books-articles/articles/transcribed-talks/buddhism-101-part-1

Figley, C.R. (2002) *Compassion Fatigue: Coping with Secondary Traumatic Stress Disorder in Those Who Treat the Traumatized.* New York: Brunner/Mazel.

Floyd, M., Rice, J. and Black, S. (2002) 'Recurrence of posttraumatic stress disorder in late life: a cognitive aging perspective.' *Journal of Clinical Geropsychology 8,* 4, 303–311.

Frazer, D.W., Hinrichsen, G.A. and Jongsma, A.E. (2014) *The Older Adult Psychotherapy Treatment Planner, with DSM-5 Updates.* New Jersey: John Wiley & Sons Inc.

Fronsdal, G. (2004) *Not-Knowing.* California: Insight Meditation Center. Accessed on 07/05/2017 at www.insightmeditationcenter.org/books-articles/articles/not-knowing

Gaddis, S. (2014) *Decentered and Influential.* Narrative Therapy Initiative, Blog: Reflecting Surfaces. Massachusetts: The Salem Center for Therapy Training and Research. Accessed on 14/06/2017 at www.narrativetherapyinitiative.org/single-post/2014/09/28/Decentered-and-Influential

Gemmel, N. (2017) *After.* New York: Harper Collins Publishing Company.

Gerfo, M.L. (1980) 'Three ways of reminiscence in theory and practice.' *The International Journal of Aging and Human Development 12,* 1, 39–48.

Goldberg, D.S. and McGee, S.J. (2011) *BMC Public Health.* United Kingdom: Pain as a Global Public Health Priority. Accessed on 19/04/2017 at https://bmcpublichealth. biomedcentral.com/articles/10.1186/1471-2458-11-770

Government of South Australia (2009) *Health Service Framework for Older People 2009–2016: Improving Health and Wellbeing Together.* South Australia: SA Health.

Haight, B.K. (1982) *Life Review and Experiencing Form.* Accessed on 16/08/2017 at http://69.195.124.63/~reminis8/wp-content/uploads/2012/12/LREF.pdf

Hall, C. (2011) *Beyond Kübler-Ross: Recent Developments in Our Understanding of Grief and Bereavement.* In-Psych publication. Melbourne: The Australian Psychological Society Limited. Accessed on 07/05/2017 at www.psychology.org.au/publications/inpsych/2011/december/hall

Harris, R. (2007) *The Happiness Trap: Stop Struggling, Start Living.* Wollombi: Exisle Publishing Limited.

Harris, R. (2009) *ACT Made Simple.* California: New Harbinger Publications Incorporated.

Heimberg, R.G. and Ritter, M.R. (2008) 'Cognitive Behavioral Therapy and Acceptance Commitment Therapy for the anxiety disorders: two approaches with much to offer.' *Clinical Psychology: Science and Practice 15,* 4, 296–298.

Helmes, E., Bird, M. and Fleming, R. (2008) 'Training for work in aged care.' *In-Psych (Special Issue on Residential Aged Care Issues) 30,* 6, 12–13.

Hill, R.D. (2008) *Seven Strategies for Positive Aging.* New York: W.W. Norton & Company.

Hitchcock, K. (2015) 'Dear life: on caring for the elderly.' *Quarterly Essay 57,* 1–78.

Hofmann, S.G. and Asmundson, G.J.G (2008) 'Acceptance and mindfulness-based therapy: new wave or old hat? *Clinical Psychology Review 28,* 1, 1–16.

Hooyman, N.R. and Kiyak, H.A. (2011) *Social Gerontology: A Multidisciplinary Perspective* (9th Ed.). Boston: Pearson Education.

Howell, C., Murphy, M. and Opolski, M. (2009) *Introduction to Interpersonal Therapy: Participant Manual.* Adelaide: CM Consulting.

Hudson P.L., Schofield P., Kelly B., Hudson R. *et al.* (2006) 'Responding to desire to die statements from patients with advanced disease: recommendations for health professionals.' *Palliative Medicine,* October, 7, 703–710.

Hummert, M.L., Garstka, T.A., Shaner, J.L. and Strahm, S. (1995) 'Judgments about stereotypes of the elderly: attitudes, age associations, and typicality ratings of young, middle-aged, and elderly adults.' *Research on Ageing 17,* 2, 168–189.

International Positive Psychology Association (2017) *Executive Committee and About IPPA.* Minnesota: International Positive Psychology Association. Accessed on 01/05/2017 at www.ippanetwork.org/about

Jonasson, J. (2015) *The Hundred-Year-Old Man Who Climbed out of the Window and Disappeared.* London: Little, Brown Book Group.

Jorm, A. and Mackinnon, A. (1995) *Psychogeriatric Assessment Scales: User's Guide* (4th Ed.). Canberra: Commonwealth Department of Health. Accessed on 04/05/2017 at https://agedcare.health.gov.au/sites/g/files/net1426/f/documents/12_2016/pas_user_guide_-_4th_edition_may_2016.pdf

Kabat-Zinn, J. (2013) *Full Catastrophe Living* (Rev. Ed.). New York: Bantam Books.

Kezelman, C. and Stavropoulos, P. (2012) *'The Last Frontier': Practice Guidelines for Treatment of Complex Trauma and Trauma Informed Care and Service Delivery.* New South Wales: Adults Surviving Childhood Abuse (now BlueKnot Foundation).

Knight, B.G. (2004) *Psychotherapy with Older Adults* (3rd Ed.). California: Sage Publications.

Knight, B.G. and Pachana, N.A. (2015) *Psychological Assessment and Therapy with Older Adults.* Oxford: Oxford University Press.

Ko, H. (2014) *Counseling Older Adults: An Asian Perspective.* Singapore: Write Editions/Tusitala (RLS) Pte Ltd.

Koder, D. and Helmes, E. (2006) 'Clinical psychologists in aged care in Australia: a question of attitude or training?' *Australian Psychologist 41,* 179–185.

Kornfield, J. (2008) *The Wise Heart: A Guide to the Universal Teachings of Buddhist Psychology.* New York: Bantam Books.

Kübler-Ross, E. (1969) *On Death and Dying.* New York: Macmillan.

Le Couteur, D.G., Bansal, A.S. and Price, D.A. (1997) 'The attitudes of medical students towards careers in geriatric medicine.' *Australian Journal on Ageing 16,* 225–228. In Australian Psychological Society (2000) *Psychology and Ageing: A Position Paper Prepared for the Australian Psychological Society by a Working Group of the Directorate of Social Issues.* Position Paper. Melbourne: The Australian Psychological Society Ltd.

Levine, P.A. and Phillips, M. (2013) *Freedom from Pain: Discover Your Body's Power to Overcome Physical Pain.* Colorado: Sounds True Inc.

Ling, J., Hunter, S.V. and Maple, M. (2014) 'Navigating the challenges of trauma counselling: how counsellors thrive and sustain their engagement.' *Australian Social Work 67,* 2, 297–310.

London, B. (1932) *Ending the Depression through Planned Obsolescence.* New York: Bernard London.

Lui, C., Warbuton, J. and Winterton, R. (2011) 'Critical reflections on a social inclusion approach for an ageing Australia.' *Australian Social Work 64,* 3, 266–282.

Mackay, H. (1997) *Generations: Baby Boomers, Their Parents and Their Children.* Sydney: Pan Macmillan Australia.

MBF Foundation (2007) *The High Price of Pain: The Economic Impact of Persistent Pain in Australia.* Sydney: Pain Management Research Institute, University of Sydney. Accessed on 16/08/2017 at www.bupa.com.au/staticfiles/BupaP3/Health%20 and%20Wellness/MediaFiles/PDFs/MBF_Foundation_the_price_of_pain.pdf

McAdams, D. (1993) *The Stories We Live by: Personal Myths and the Making of Self.* New York: The Guilford Press.

McCormack, B. (2003) 'A conceptual framework for person-centred practice with older people.' *International Journal of Nursing Practice 9,* 3, 202–209.

Misrachi, S. (2012) 'Lives Unseen: Unacknowledged Trauma of Non-Disordered, Competent Adult Children of Parents with a Severe Mental Illness (ACOPSMI).' Masters research thesis, Department of Social Work, Melbourne School of Health Sciences, The University of Melbourne.

Misrachi, S. (2015) 'Do no harm: 11 reasons why we shouldn't rely on 'Stages' as a grief model.' *Mind Café 15,* 9.

Moore, S.L., Metcalf, B. and Schow, E. (2000) 'Aging and meaning in life: examining the concept.' *Geriatric Nursing 21,* 1, 27–29.

Morgan, A. (ed.) (1999) *Once upon a Time...: Narrative Therapy with Children and Their Families.* South Australia: Dulwich Centre Publications.

Moseley, L. and Butler, D. (2015) *The Explain Pain Handbook: Protectometer.* Adelaide: Noigroup Publications.

Myerhoff, B. (1976) *Number Our Days.* Video documentary. United States: Loring d'Usseau, Lynne Littman and Barbara Myerhoff.

Myerhoff, B. (1982) 'Life History among the Elderly: Performance, Visibility, and Re-membering.' In J. Ruby (ed.) *A Crack in the Mirror: Reflective Perspectives in Anthropology.* Pennsylvania: University of Pennsylvania Press.

Myerhoff, B. (1986) '"Life Not Death in Venice": Its Second Life.' In V. Turner and E. Bruner (eds) *The Anthropology of Experience.* Chicago: University of Illinois Press.

O'Donoghue, M. (2011) 'Teaching meditation 3: loving-kindness.' *Journal of the Australian and New Zealand Student Services Association,* October, 38, 15–21.

Office for National Statistics (2013) *What Does the 2011 Census Tell Us about Older People.* United Kingdom: Office for National Statistics. Accessed on 15/04/2017 at www. ons.gov.uk/peoplepopulationandcommunity/birthsdeathsandmarriages/ageing/ articles/whatdoesthe2011censustellusaboutolderpeople/2013-09-06

Ogden, P. (2012) 'Beyond Conversation in Sensorimotor Psychotherapy: Embedded Relational Mindfulness.' In V.M. Follette, D. Rozelle, J.W. Hopper, D.I. Rome and J. Briere (eds) *Contemplative Methods in Trauma Management: Integrating Mindfulness and Other Approaches.* New York: The Guilford Press.

Oliver, M. (2010) *Evidence.* Boston: Beacon Press.

Pachana, N.A. (2008) 'Psychologists' role in enhancing care in residential aged care facilities: current issues, future directions.' *In-Psych (Special Issue on Residential Aged Care Issues) 30,* 6, 8–11.

Pachana, N.A. (2013) *Geropsychology Workforce Crisis: An International Perspective.* Milwaukee: Bulletin of the International Psychogeriatrics Association. Accessed on 07/05/2017 at www.ipa-online.org/about-ipa/ipa-news-and-media/workforce-issues/geropsychology-workforce-crisis-an-international-perspective

Pachana, N. (2016) *Ageing: A Very Short Introduction.* Oxford: Oxford University Press.

Pachana, N., Byrne, G., Siddle, H., Koloski, N., Harley, E. and Arnold, E. (2007) 'Development and validation of the Geriatric Anxiety Inventory.' *International Psychogeriatrics 19,* 1, 103–114.

Pachana, N.A., Helmes, E., Byrne, G.J.A., Edelstein, B.A., Konnert, C.A. and Pot, A.M. (2010) 'Screening for mental disorders in residential aged care facilities.' *International Psychogeriatrics 22*, 7, 1107–1120.

Pachana, N., Helmes, E. and Koder D.A. (2006) 'Guidelines for the provision of psychological services for older adults.' *Australian Psychologist 41*, 1, 15–22.

Pain Australia (2017a) *Campaign for Pain.* Sydney: Pain Australia. Accessed on 20/10/2017 at www.painaustralia.org.au/static/uploads/files/campaignforpainbriefingkit-jul-2016 -wfwqkfaatitr.pdf

Pain Australia (2017b) *Older People and Those Living With a Disability.* Sydney: Pain Australia. Accessed on 16/08/2017 at www.painaustralia.org.au/about-pain/who-it-affects/older-people-those-living-with-a-disability

Pilotlight Australia (2007) *Dying to Know: Bringing Death to Life.* Melbourne: Pilotlight Australia.

Pursey, A., and Luker, K. (1995) 'Attitudes and stereotypes: nurses' work with older people.' *Journal of Advanced Nursing 22*, 547–555. In Australian Psychological Society (2000) *Psychology and Ageing: A Position Paper Prepared for the Australian Psychological Society by a Working Group of the Directorate of Social Issues.* Position Paper. Melbourne: The Australian Psychological Society Ltd.

Rider, K., Gallagher-Thompson, D. and Thompson, L. (2004) *California Older Person's Pleasant Events Schedule: Manual.* California: Rider, Gallagher-Thompson and Thompson. Accessed on 05/05/2017 at http://oafc.stanford.edu/coppes_files/Manual2.pdf

Rothschild, B. (2000) *The Body Remembers: The Psychophysiology of Trauma and Trauma Treatment.* New York: W.W. Norton & Company.

Rogers, C. (1995) *A Way of Being.* New York: Houghton Mifflin Company.

Royal Australian and New Zealand College of Psychiatrists (2010) *Older Australians Deserve a Better Deal in Mental Health.* Victoria: Royal Australian and New Zealand College of Psychiatrists. Accessed on 17/04/2017 at www.ranzcp.org/Files/Resources/Older_Australians_Deserve_a_Better_Deal_in_Mental_.aspx

Royal Australian and New Zealand College of Psychiatrists (2015) *Position Statement No. 22: Psychiatry Services for Older People.* Victoria: Royal Australian and New Zealand College of Psychiatrists. Accessed on 29/06/2017 at www.ranzcp.org/Files/Resources/College_Statements/Position_Statements/PS-22-FPOA-Psychiatry-services-for-older-peopl-(1).aspx

Russell, S. (2017) Personal communication, 15 June.

Schore, A. (2012) *The Science of the Art of Psychotherapy.* New York: W.W. Norton & Company.

Scogin, F. (2009) *Depression and Suicide in Older Adults Resource Guide.* Washington: American Psychological Association. Accessed on 11/06/2017 at www.apa.org/pi/aging/resources/guides/depression.aspx

Secker, D.L., Kazantzis, N. and Pachana, N.A. (2004) 'Cognitive behaviour for older adults: guidelines for adapting therapy structure. *Journal of Rational-Emotive and Cognitive-Behavioural Therapy 22*, 2, 93–109.

Segal, D.L., Honn Qualls, S. and Smyer, M.A. (2010) *Aging and Mental Health: Second Edition.* Brisbane: John Wiley and Sons Ltd, Wiley-Blackwell (an imprint of John Wiley & Sons Ltd).

Segal, Z.V., Williams, J.M.G. and Teasdale, J.D. (2002) *Mindfulness-Based Cognitive Therapy for Depression: A New Approach to Preventing Relapse* (1st Ed.). New York: The Guilford Press.

Siegel, D.J. (2010) *Mindsight: The New Science of Personal Transformation.* New York: Bantam Books.

Smith, B. (2016) *Sex in Aged Care Facilities Shunned and Prevented Says Study.* Armidale: The University of New England. Accessed on 06/05/2017 at https://blog.une.edu.au/news/2016/06/22/sex-in-aged-care-facilities-shunned-and-prevented-says-study/

Snowdon, J. (1997) 'Depression in old age: questions concerning prevalence studies.' *International Journal of Geriatric Psychiatry 12,* 1043–1045. In Australian Psychological Society (2000) *Psychology and Ageing: A Position Paper Prepared for the Australian Psychological Society by a Working Group of the Directorate of Social Issues.* Position Paper. Melbourne: The Australian Psychological Society Ltd.

Stamm, B.H. (2002) 'Measuring Compassion Satisfaction As Well As Fatigue: Developmental History of the Compassion Fatigue and Satisfaction Test.' In C.R. Figley (ed.) *Treating Compassion Fatigue* (pp.107–119). New York: Brunner/Mazel.

Steury, S. and Blank, M. (1977) *Readings In Psychotherapy with Older People* (DHEW Publication ADM 77-409). Washington, DC: Government Printing Office. In B.G. Knight (2004) *Psychotherapy with Older Adults* (3rd Ed.). California: Sage Publications.

Stroebe, M. and Schut, H. (2010) 'The dual process model of coping with bereavement: a decade on.' *Omega 61,* 4, 273–289.

Sween, E. (1998) 'The one minute question: What is narrative therapy?' *Gecko 2,* 3–6.

Swisher, A.K. (2010) 'Practice-based evidence.' *Cardiopulmonary Physical Therapy Journal 21,* 2, 4.

Tedeschi, R.G. and Calhoun, L.G. (1995) *Trauma and Transformation: Growing in the Aftermath of Suffering.* California: Sage Publishing.

Tedeschi, R.G. and Calhoun, L.G. (2004) 'The foundations of posttraumatic growth: new considerations.' *Psychological Inquiry 15,* 1–18. doi:10.1207/s15327965pli1501_01.

Tanner, D. and Harris, J. (2008) *Working with Older People.* New York: Routledge.

Tipping, S.A. and Whiteside, M. (2015) 'Language reversion among people with dementia from culturally and linguistically diverse backgrounds: the family experience.' *Australian Social Work 68,* 2, 184–197.

Tonkin, T. (2013) Personal communication, 27 April.

Transgenerational Design Matters (2017) *The Demographics of Aging: Characteristics of our Aging Population.* New Mexico: Transgenerational Design Matters. Accessed on 15/10/2017 at http://transgenerational.org/aging/demographics.htm

United Nations (2002) *World Population Ageing 1950–2050.* New York: United Nations Department of Economic and Social Affairs Population Division.

UniThrive (2016) *Introduction to Meditation by Mark O'Donoghue.* The Practice of Meditation, UniThrive video series. Adelaide: University of Adelaide. Accessed on 04/06/2017 at www.adelaide.edu.au/uni-thrive/engage/meditation

University of Leicester (2017) *Emotion Thermometers Tool.* Leicester: University of Leicester. Accessed on 05/05/2017 at www.psycho-oncology.info/ET.htm

Walser, R.D. and Westrup, D. (2007) *Acceptance and Commitment Therapy for the Treatment of Post-Traumatic Stress Disorder and Trauma-Related Problems: A Practitioner's Guide to Using Mindfulness and Acceptance Strategies.* California: New Harbinger Publications Incorporated.

Wells, Y., Bhar, S., Kinsella, G., Kowalski, C. *et al.* (2014) *What Works to Promote Emotional Wellbeing in Older People: A Guide for Aged Care Staff Working in Community or Residential Care Settings.* Melbourne: Beyondblue.

White, M. (1992) 'Deconstruction and therapy.' In *Experience, Contradiction, Narrative and Imagination: Selected papers of David Epston and Michael White 1989–1991.* Adelaide: Dulwich Centre Publications.

White, M. (1998) 'Saying "Hullo" Again: The Incorporation of the Lost Relationship in the Resolution of Grief.' In C. White and D. Denborough (eds) *Introducing Narrative Therapy: A Collection of Practice-Based Writings.* Adelaide: Dulwich Centre Publications.

White, M. (2005) *Workshop Notes.* Adelaide: Dulwich Centre Publications. Accessed on 11/06/2017 at www.dulwichcentre.com.au/michael-white-workshop-notes.pdf

White, M. and Epston, D. (1989) *Literate Means to Therapeutic Ends.* Adelaide: Dulwich Centre Publications.

Whyte, J. (2013) Personal communication, 14 November.

Whyte, J. (2017) Personal communication, 1 June.

Wilde, O. (1894) 'Phrases and Philosophies for the Use of the Young.' *The Chameleon,* December edition.

Yesavage, J.A. (1988) 'Geriatric Depression Scale (short version).' *Psychopharmacology Bulletin 24,* 4, 709–711.

Yesavage, J.A., Brink, T.L., Rose, T.L., Lum, O. *et al.* (1983) 'Development and validation of a geriatric depression screening scale: a preliminary report.' *Journal of Psychiatric Research 17,* 37–49.

Zisook, S. and Downs, N.S. (1998) 'Diagnosis and treatment of depression in late life.' *Journal of Clinical Psychiatry 59,* 4, 80–91. In Australian Psychological Society (2000) *Psychology and Ageing: A Position Paper Prepared for the Australian Psychological Society by a Working Group of the Directorate of Social Issues.* Position Paper. Melbourne: The Australian Psychological Society Ltd.

Presentations and workshops

Bogenberger, R.P. (2014) 'Aging and mental health: assessment, treatment and management. Video workshop.' Facilitated by the Psychology and Health Forum, Adelaide.

Frallch, T. (2012) 'Advanced mindfulness: integrating cutting-edge neuroscience and mindfulness skills in the treatment of mental health disorders and emotional dysregulation.' Video workshop, facilitated by TATRA.

Kessler, D. (2015) 'Grief, complicated grief, divorce, breakup and other losses, participatory workshop.' Facilitated by TATRA, Adelaide.

Neimeyer, R. (2000) 'Meaning reconstruction and the experience of loss.' Facilitated by the Centre for Grief Education, Adelaide.

White, M. (2000) 'Level One Intensive.' Facilitated by the Dulwich Centre, Adelaide.

Whyte, J., Pachana, N. and McKay, R. (2012) 'Collaborative care for older people with mental health issues.' Webinar facilitated by the Mental Health Professionals Network, Australia. Accessed on 02/08/2017 at www.mhpn.org.au/WebinarRecording/28/Collaborative-care-for-older-people-with-mental-health-issues#.WXsPfVFLflU

Further Reading and Resources

Baker, A.E.Z and Procter, N.G. (2013) 'A qualitative inquiry into consumer beliefs about the cause of mental illness.' *Journal of Psychiatric and Mental Health Nursing 20*, 442–447.

Chapman, S.A. (2005) 'Theorizing about aging well: constructing a narrative.' *Canadian Journal on Aging 24*, 1, 9–18.

Chochinov, H.M. (2004) 'Dignity and the eye of the beholder.' *Journal of Clinical Oncology 22*, 7, 1336–1340.

Egan, G. (1990) *The Skilled Helper: A Systematic Approach to Effective Helping* (4th Ed.). California: Brooks/Cole Publishing Company.

Gamble, T.K. and Gamble M. (1993) *Communication Works* (4th Ed.). New York: McGraw-Hill Inc.

Howell, C. (2007) *Keeping The Blues Away: A Guide to Reducing the Relapse of Depression.* Adelaide: ARI Pty. Ltd.

Kadushin, A. and Kadushin G. (1997) *The Social Work Interview: A Guide for Human Service Professionals* (4th Ed.). United States of America: Columbia University Press.

McDonald, P.A. and Haney, M. (1997) *Counseling The Older Adult: A Training Manual in Clinical Gerontology.* California: Jossey-Bass.

McInnis-Dittrich, K. (2009) 'Working with Older Adults Support Systems: Spouses, Partners, Families and Caregivers.' In *Social Work With Older Adults: A Biopsychosocial Approach to Assessment and Intervention* (3rd Ed.) Boston: Pearson.

McKay, M., Davis, M. and Fanning, P. (1983) *Messages: The Communication Skills Book.* California: New Harbinger Publications.

Molzahn, A.E. (2007) 'Spirituality in later life: effect on quality of life.' *Journal of Gerontological Nursing 33*, 1, 32–39.

O'Connell, B. (2012) 'The First Session.' In *Solution-focused Therapy* (3rd Ed.) (pp.39–76). Los Angeles: Sage.

Randall, W.L. and Kenyon, G.M. (2004) 'Time, story, and wisdom: emerging themes in narrative gerontology.' *Canadian Journal on Aging 23*, 4, 334–346.

Shilson, K. (2014) *Sensorimotor Psychotherapy.* Canada: InsideOut Psychological Services. Accessed on 21/06/2017 at www.insideoutpsych.ca/sensorimotor-psychotherapy

The Council of State Governments (2012) *Policies and Programs to Help America's Senior Citizens.* USA. Accessed on 15/04/17 at http://knowledgecenter.csg.org/kc/content/policies-and-programs-help-america%E2%80%99s-senior-citizens

Walser, R.D. (2016) Ph.D. TL Consultation Services Mindfulness Information. Adapted from: *Acceptance and Commitment Therapy for Depression in Veterans* by Robyn D. Walser, Katie Sears, Maggie Chartier and Bradly Karlin (workshop handout Adelaide).

White, C. and Hales, J. (eds "collected by") *The Personal is the Professional: Therapists Reflect on Their Families, Lives and Work.* Adelaide: Dulwich Publications.

Resources for the United States of America

The Friendship Line at the Institute on Aging: 800.971.0016
   www.ioaging.org/services/all-inclusive-health-care/friendship-line
   A 24-hour crisis support service that assists with:

- active suicide intervention

- providing emotional support

- elder abuse prevention and counselling

- giving wellbeing checks

- grief support through assistance and reassurance

- information and referrals for isolated older adults, and adults living with disabilities.

Resources for Australia

Lifeline: 13 11 14
   www.lifeline.org.au
   A 24-hour crisis support and suicide prevention.
My Aged Care: 1800 200 422
   www.myagedcare.gov.au
   The entry point for aged care services and information.

Resources for the United Kingdom

The Silver Line: 0800 4 70 80 90
   www.thesilverline.org.uk
   A 24-hour helpline providing information, friendship and advice to older people.

Notes

1. Despite the fact that geropsychology has been a field of research in America for decades, it was only in 2010 that professional geropsychology became a specialty of psychology under the American Psychological Association.
2. The AASW would like to note that it is not compulsory for members to provide them with data regarding their field of practice and members may change fields of practice without updating their membership record.
3. A Senate Enquiry reveals that older Australians are expecting better quality from the aged care workforce (www.australianageingagenda.com.au/2016/11/09/peaks-raise-aged-care-staffing-levels-and-skills-mix-with-senate-inquiry) and American geropsychologist Bob G. Knight predicts that as Baby Boomers age, the need and demand for mental health services will increase (www.apa.org/pi/aging/resources/guides/psychotherapy.aspx).
4. See for example: *Psychological Assessment and Therapy with Older Adults* by Bob G. Knight and Nancy A. Pachana (2015); *The Older Adult Psychotherapy Treatment Planner, with DSM-5 Updates* by Deborah W. Frazer, Gregory A. Hinrichsen and Arthur E. Jongsma (2014); *Counseling Older Adults* by John Blando (2014); *Counseling Older Adults: An Asian Perspective* by Helen Ko (2014); and *Aging and Mental Health* by Daniel L. Segal, Sara Honn Qualls and Michael A. Smyer (2010).
5. With an ageing population there is now increasing awareness to address elder abuse. The United Nations General Assembly has designated 15 June as World Elder Abuse Awareness Day. See their website link at www.un.org/en/events/elderabuse.
6. In Australia there are multiple report lines depending on the State or Territory. Where I live, South Australia, it is the Aged Rights Advocacy Service. In the United States it is the National Center on Elder Abuse, in the United Kingdom it is Action on Elder Abuse and the United Nations has a World Elder Abuse Awareness Day every year on 15 June.
7. See Chapter 4 for a description of the Mini Mental State Examination.
8. The term "persistent pain" is preferred now amongst health professionals and pain management specialists compared to "chronic pain". The reason for this is because chronic pain can relate to unhelpful expectations that the condition is able to be cured – thus creating a psychological barrier for patients in their ability to explore ways to live with their pain in a manageable way and accepting that it is not able to be cured. Therefore in this book I will refer to "persistent pain" and not "chronic pain".
9. Please note that delirium can be experienced as either hypo or hyper presentations and that this table does not describe all the variances that can be noted on this continuum.

10. Please note that, for the sake of simplicity, grief in this description more typifies "normal" grief and not "complicated grief" – see "grief" in the definitions section at the back of this book for a fuller description on the range of presentations.

11. Not always associated with death – any loss that is a primary, secondary or tertiary loss.

12. You can download the Emotion Thermometers handout at www.psycho-oncology. info/ET.htm

13. The author would like to acknowledge Professor McAdams's process of the same title, which can be found at www.sesp.northwestern.edu/docs/Interviewrevised95.pdf

14. The "Some Experiences of Grief" handout is included in Appendix 3 of this book.

15. The Dual Process Model of Coping with Bereavement is a model representing human grief and is designed by Margaret Stroebe and Henk Schut (2010) who suggest that managing bereavement requires a combination of confronting it (a focus on loss) and accepting it (a focus on restoration). It can be very useful for people to understand the triggers and meaning making in their grief story/stories. An image of it can be found here: www.google.com.au/search?q=The+Dual+Process+Model+of+Coping +with+Bereavement&client=firefox-b-ab&source=lnms&tbm=isch&sa=X&ved=0a hUKEwjw7NH8u8fUAhUGbbwKHbt-BgEQ_AUICigB&biw=1366&bih=610#im grc=Wrbt08Ls-76PNM

16. Please refer again to note 8.

17. Loving-kindness is a specific kind of love conceptualized in various religious traditions, both among theologians and religious practitioners, as a form of love characterized by acts of kindness.

18. For an explanation of the limbic system please see the definition section at the back of this book.

19. The Anchor Activity or Dropping the Anchor is an activity cited in *ACT Made Simple* (Harris 2009, pp.166–167) which asks clients to combine a focus on the breath with gently pushing both feet into the floor to contact with the present moment.

20. Currently evidence-based treatments supported by Veterans Affairs for PTSD include Prolonged Exposure Therapy and Cognitive Processing Therapy (Cook and Wiltsey Stirman 2015) and Acceptance and Commitment Therapy is increasingly being used with a veteran population (Walser and Westrup 2007).

21. This is a term that is used in geropsychology but it is not one that I personally use because of how much it appears to privilege a therapist's view about "right or wrong", appears weighted to the negative, and because I favour intervention that seeks not to change thought content but relate to it differently.

22. Stolen Generations or Stolen Children are terms given to honour the forcible removal of Aboriginal and Torres Strait Islander children from their families by the Australian government which took place between 1905 and 1969.

23. See the following articles and petition: www.smh.com.au/national/health/nursing-homes-story-headline-20161228-gtiqc6.html and www.abc.net.au/news/2017-01-17/most-nursing-home-residents-denied-psychological-care/8186546 and healthforolderaustralians.org.au

Subject Index

Author Index